Health Essentials

Naturopathy

Stewart Mitchell BPhil, an experienced clinician and trainer, studied naturopathy in the UK, India and the USA. He is in private practice and directs the School of Complementary Therapies in Exeter, southern England. He also conducts training programmes for the UK National Health Service. He combines this with operating The Cafe, an outdoor restaurant which encourages relaxed, healthy eating. He holds a research degree in Complementary Health Studies from the University of Exeter.

He is also the author of *Massage – A Practical Introduction* (Element 1992) and *The Complete Illustrated Guide to Massage* (Element 1997)

The Health Essentials Series

There is a growing number of people who find themselves attracted to holistic or alternative therapies and natural approaches to maintaining optimum health and vitality. The *Health Essentials* series is designed to help the newcomer by presenting high quality introductions to all the main complementary health subjects. Each book presents all the essential information on each therapy, explaining what it is, how it works and what it can do for the reader. Advice is also given, where possible, on how to begin using the therapy at home, together with comprehensive lists of courses and classes available worldwide.

The *Health Essentials* titles are all written by practising experts in their fields. Exceptionally clear and concise, each text is supported by attractive illustrations.

Series Medical Consultant
Dr John Cosh MD, FRCP

In the same series
Acupressure by Richard Brennan
Acupuncture by Peter Mole
Alexander Technique by Richard Brennan
Aromatherapy by Christine Wildwood
Ayurveda by Scott Gerson
Chi Kung by James MacRitchie
Chinese Medicine by Tom Williams
Colour Therapy by Pauline Wills
Flower Remedies by Christine Wildwood
Herbal Medicine by Vicki Pitman
Homeopathy by Peter Adams
Iridology by John and Sheelagh Colton
Kinesiology by Ann Holdway
Massage by Stewart Mitchell
Natural Beauty by Sidra Shaukat
Reflexology by Inge Dougans with Suzanne Ellis
Self-Hypnosis by Elaine Sheehan
Shiatsu by Elaine Liechti
Spiritual Healing by Jack Angelo
Vitamin Guide by Hasnain Walji

NATUROPATHY

Understanding the Healing Power of Nature

STEWART MITCHELL

E L E M E N T
Shaftesbury, Dorset • Boston, Massachusetts
Melbourne, Victoria

© Element Books Limited 1998
Text © Stewart Mitchell 1998

First published in Great Britain in 1998 by
Element Books Limited
Shaftesbury, Dorset SP7 8BP

Published in the USA in 1998 by
Element Books Inc.
160 North Washington Street,
Boston, Massachusetts 02114

Published in Australia in 1998 by
Element Books and distributed by
Penguin Australia Limited
487 Maroondah Highway,
Ringwood, Victoria 3134

Cover design by Slatter-Anderson
Cover photography by J. Cat Photography
Design by Roger Lightfoot
Typeset by Footnote Graphics
Printed and bound in Great Britain by
Biddles Ltd, Guildford & King's Lynn

British Library Cataloguing in Publication
data available

Library of Congress Cataloging in Publication
data available

ISBN 1 86204 303 5

Note from the Publisher

Any information given in any book in the *Health Essentials* series is
not intended to be taken as a replacement for medical advice. Any
person with a condition requiring medical attention should consult a
qualified medical practitioner or suitable therapist.

Contents

List of Figures   vi

Introduction   1

1 The Development of Naturopathy   7

2 The Principles of Naturopathy   17

3 Naturopathy in Practice   26

4 How Naturopathic Treatment Works   46

5 Naturopathic Care for Adults   72

6 Naturopathic Care of Children   93

7 Naturopathic First Aid   100

8 Taking Naturopathy Further   115

Appendix: The Personagram   120

Glossary   124

Recommended Reading   128

Useful Addresses   130

Index   132

List of Figures

Figure 1	The insignia of Asclepius	8
Figure 2	The Alexander Technique	34
Figure 3	The digestive system	53
Figure 4	Practise hatha yoga	54
Figure 5	The human skeleton	58
Figure 6	Self-massage for the neck region	59
Figure 7	Professional treatment for relaxation	63
Figure 8	The lymphatic system	65
Figure 9	The brain, showing relative structures	68
Figure 10	Activating the vagus nerves	69
Figure 11	Exercise with movements that involve arm-raising	76
Figure 12	A birth pool	80
Figure 13	Beginning graduated physical exercise	83
Figure 14	The recovery position	87
Figure 15	Cross section of a joint	90
Figure 16	Indulge in a tantrum	92
Figure 17	A compress	103
Figure 18	The layers of the skin	108

To Gilli

Introduction

Sickness is not just an isolated event, nor an unfortunate brush with nature. It is a form of communication – the language of the organs – through which nature, society and culture speak simultaneously. The individual body should be seen as the most immediate, the proximate terrain where social truths and social contradictions are played out, as well as a locus of personal resistance, creativity and change.

Nancy Scheper-Hughes and Margaret M Lock
University of California, Berkley & McGill University

OUR HEALTH IS CONCERNED with the quality of life as much as its duration. We know that we must survive, but we must also be able to enjoy. A comprehensive definition of health may be elusive, but being well is an inner sensation; an awareness that not only because of, but sometimes in spite of, our circumstances, we are *well*.

Feelings of uneasiness or disorder do not threaten wellness completely but beyond a certain point symptoms of strain begin to appear. In the modern world, we take it for granted that it is the role of our health-care systems to respond at such times until inner composure, homeostatis, is re-established. Comparatively recently in the evolution of human beings, a system of care developed whose therapeutic aim is the annihilation of symptoms. Its influence is so persuasive that it is now the conventional treatment of disorders world-wide. This system is popularly called 'modern medicine'.

The modern method is based on the assumption that symptoms represent virulant attacks from without, and a massed

1

array of medicines, vaccines and surgical procedures are directed against the perceived externalized agencies of ill-health. Because of its contention that illness is a condition of the physical body, the conventional method is also known as 'biomedicine'.

Another approach, which predates conventional health care, interprets illness in a wider context. It prefers to work alongside symptoms, using them as a guide to treatments which will raise the health profile of the individual; this method is called naturopathy.

Well-being is influenced by many factors – personal, social, educational and economic – and we would be mistaken to regard any system of care as more than part of a complicated picture of health in which therapies and personal circumstances interact.

The role of biomedicine has been largely technological. As well as pharmaceutical armoury, it has also developed sophisticated methods of detecting and treating disorders. At a microbiological level its impressive achievements include work with complex genetic and metabolic conditions, and it has greatly improved our chances of surviving accidental trauma. But the general application of biomedicine has not seen widespread success. Having played its part in eradicating the disorders of the impoverished preceding centuries, it is becoming increasingly ineffective in addressing the rise of major health problems in present times – the so-called 'lifestyle' disorders.

Attention has also been drawn to the unwanted side-effects of certain biomedical treatments, which have created new medical conditions. This development contributes to an increasingly recognized problem of extending care along biomedical lines: its technology is becoming so expensive to provide that it may become financially impossible to continue to deliver therapeutically, even at its present level.

In contrast, naturopathy is low-tech, low-cost and its treatments are collaborative, so that care begins as a joint responsibility, which is ultimately assumed by the patient. It has been said that the former disorders of poverty and misery have been replaced by those associated with plenty and discontent. Naturopathic methods are very relevant to the treatment of these illnesses, which are increasingly and fatally affecting people's lives in affluent Western societies.

Naturopathy's basic tenet is that human life is governed by the same self-regulating, self-repairing forces that care for all living things. This holds for everyone – children, adults and older individuals – except in extreme circumstances associated with malnutrition. Treatment consists in interpreting symptoms so as to release inhibitions on the self-regulating mechanisms and provide relief from discomfort and distress. Its methods are natural in that they utilize readily available resources such as food, touch and water, but do not require specific products.

Naturopathy is strictly scientific, seeing every manifestation of disorder as the result of an understandable cause, or more likely several causes. It has a mystical aspect, but not in the direct application of treatment. Rather, it manifests itself in respect for the way treatment is complemented by the unknowable, immeasurable healing force within all life.

The rationale for naturopathy is also taken from the experiences of individuals who have survived without the benefit of conventional medicine. In our evolution, this means the vast majority of human beings who have ever lived. There are few detailed records of the health of ancient people except what can be inferred from the study of still existing primitive communities who have been unaffected by modernity, but apparently, our ancient forebears led a relatively stress-free and leisurely existence, unmolested in the main by monstrous creatures. It is suggested from scraps of evidence that their day was effortless in comparison with ours and it is estimated that earlier human beings spent very little time 'working' at life. Perhaps aware of this prehistoric rhythm at some deep level, a colleague once related her typical week: two days at her job; one day to do personal jobs; one day for creativity; one day exclusively devoted to her daughter; one day for the unexpected; leaving one day . . . off!

There are still in the world today communities who have retained the customs of early human beings – not those exotic Shangri-las of health-food fantasies but a few remaining people who follow the way of life known as 'hunter-gathering'. It is true that their numbers are dwindling but it is important to say that this is not because the people themselves are dying out; rather they are disadvantaged by encroaching modern technology.

Research on the !Kung people – also called the Bushpeople – of the inhospitable Kalahari Desert in Africa provides useful material to consider. Although we might imagine hunter-gathering to be of the distant past, it would be fairer to say that contemporary human beings are very much the newcomers. This so-called unsophisticated way of life is roughly one million years old – modern lifestyles are merely a veneer of 1 per cent in the timescale of human existence. It is not unreasonable, therefore, in examining what might make for a healthy lifestyle, to assume that the 'primitive' ways of our forebears have been very successful.

We might imagine that Bushpeople endure a somewhat harsh existence, yet they enjoy a life of relative leisure. Residing in the middle of an inhospitable desert region, they are free from the disturbing complications of modern technology. If they do not die prematurely from accidents, they have a good life expectancy: without the medical assistance available to Westerners, seven per cent of the population of Bushpeople were found to be over 65 years of age.

Findings on the life of the Bushpeople are interesting when contrasted with modern life. For example:

- Breastfeeding continues for up to four years – only a minority of mothers breastfeed after six months in the West.
- They have slightly worn but not carious (bad) teeth – even with access to dentistry, one-third of the present-day adult population of Glasgow, Scotland have *no teeth at all*.
- The majority of foods in their diet are sourced from vegetables. Meat is obtained infrequently from small, lean animals. Despite an often sparse if mixed diet, they showed no clinical sign of deficiency of any vitamin – contemporary urban dwellers presently spend millions per year on vitamin supplements.
- Their blood pressure falls with increasing age in men – high pressure (hypertension), which is a main contributor to heart disease, is accepted as part of the ageing process in the West. Bushpeople do not consume salt, a food additive which is linked to high blood pressure.
- Hunter-gatherers do not regard an individual's illness as an isolated experience but as connected to events within the family or wider community.

Although certain of the Bushpeople's habits have received attention within biomedical circles, the last finding – that symptoms are not exclusively of the physical body – is only beginning to be explored. Psychologists who follow the Systems

Theory of behaviour are aware that the emotional symptoms of one member of the family may be serving to release the pressure within the family as a whole. As yet, biomedicine is reluctant to make this connection with physical manifestations of disorder.

Naturopathy does not encourage self-obsession by extending the focus on symptoms to the whole of the patient's life. It is a positive attention, guided by the symptoms, which already may be causing the patient concern. Naturopaths observe that the awareness of personal needs, however confronting, is more likely to lead to a healthy outcome than ignorance or suppression.

Similarly, health is popularly described in terms of achievement and preservation but naturopathy suspects that striving for bodily health alone is illusory. Loss of health often succeeds other losses in life, which may be irreplaceable. These situations are destined to contribute to a breakdown of health unless a wider image is embraced which acknowledges the impact of social and emotional life on well-being. Naturopathy offers a practical, well-founded approach to life's problems rather than promising a hermetically sealed state of health. Its unique contribution is in offering ways in which an individual can be helped to recognize and use their situation, as dramatically presented by symptoms, to lead a more realistic, integrated life.

HOW TO USE THIS BOOK

The aim of this book is to explain naturopathy to two audiences. The first is readers who are suffering disorders, personally or within the family and, finding the rationale of naturopathy appealing, are inspired to take up its methods. It seeks to transform fears about illnesses into optimism, and divert a craving for cure into the realization that the answer is *care*.

The second audience consists of those who are biomedically inclined but not totally convinced, and who may be parents or health professionals. Naturopathy need not – in fact *should* not – be adopted wholesale, and it is possible that without first-hand knowledge of its benefits, some aspects may be regarded as unacceptable to some new readers. It is not a converting philosophy, because its appeal is primarily to an individual's intuition, being confirmed through positive experiences. An appreciation of treatment methods, impressive though they are, is really secondary to entertaining naturopathy's central theme – that symptoms are friends not enemies of health, signposts to a way of helping which is both appropriate and compassionate. Starting from where you are now, include a little naturopathy and observe what happens.

In chapter 1 of the book you will read about the background to naturopathy and its development. Chapters 2 and 3 give fundamental information about its methods, then a gently technical chapter 4 places it in its physiological context. Chapters 5 and 6 give descriptions of generalized naturopathy for commonly experienced disorders. The scope in a book this size is obviously limited but the examples given show the style of consultation and treatment a reader might expect from a practitioner.

Chapter 7 is the most practical, immediately translatable part of the book. It details hydrotherapy first aids and their usefulness in many circumstances.

All the case histories given in this book report successful treatment. This is not to suggest the infallibility of naturopathic consultation. Treatment is not known to complicate a condition but there are, of course, occasions where outcomes are less effective. The cases illustrate situations where treatment is shown to be consistently beneficial.

Chapter 8 suggests three ways of taking naturopathy further. I am happy to offer any additional help if any reader wishes to contact me at the School of Complementary Therapies in Exeter.

The Appendix offers a variant on the popular health questionnaire. It is a format which practitioners may use directly or have a patient work on at home. It offers a sensitive insight into the energies behind symptoms and a creative way of initiating change.

For the sake of fluidity, there are no references. However, titles in the lengthy Recommended Reading section contain a fuller discussion on most of the topics raised in this book. I especially recommend the writings of C Leslie Thomson and Alec Milne, Dr Robert Mendelsohn and works by Nancy Scheper-Hughes and Margaret Lock.

1

The Development of Naturopathy

Physician, at the bedside of patient who is attached to massive technological equipment: 'Nothing to worry about Mr Jones, that bleeping sound you hear is Nature's way of telling us that something is wrong.'

ORIGINS

NATUROPATHY HAS EXISTED since the days of Hippocrates. It represents the complementary view of practitioners who work within the tradition of Hygieia, the Ancient Greek goddess of health: that health is normal, life lived to the full in harmony with one's nature, and that ill-health is not caused by the interference and actions of an external entity but comes as a reminder to oneself to live a more harmonious life. The importance of health promotion combined in the early Greek system with the essential treatment of illness characterizes a tension in health care which has existed up to the present day.

Naturopathy's development has benefited from observation of nature as opposed to experimentation. It uses biologically based methods for health promotion, using diet, posture, massage and water therapy. Individual development is encouraged, with equal stress on the importance of relationships. Social awareness and responsibility towards the environment are balanced by a perspective on the human's place in the universal order.

The word naturopathy is a Latin–Greek hybrid which can be defined as 'being close to or benefiting from nature'. It is a philosophy as much as a system of health care, founded on trust in the natural order of life and the self-regulating potential of human nature. The ancient cultures of the world were founded on close co-operation with nature and had sophisticated, integrated health philosophies. In India, for example, the indigenous medicine, known as Ayurveda, is translated as 'science of life'. Central to the Chinese system of health is the concept of chi, the universal energy which is described as permeating and governing all levels of being.

Western medicine inherited twin Greek-derived systems, one of which has come to dominate illness-treating attitudes around the world. But for the early Greeks, their two approaches to health were complementary. One school of thought was naturopathic, regarding health as the norm, an entitlement from living intelligently, represented in the feminine energy of the goddess Hygieia. The other maintained, sceptically, that life's imperfection was manifest in diseases, which had to be corrected by 'doctoring'. This interventionist approach was championed in the name of the male deity, Asclepius.

While the two worked in harmony for the Greeks, it was the Asclepian way that became the predominant theme of Western health care, as evidence by his insignia on the modern medical

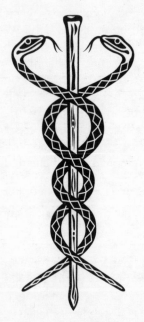

Figure 1   The insignia of Asclepius

doctor's prescription pad. Largely because of this and the prevalence of religious attitudes which denigrated the body, Westerners have not had the benefit of naturopathy until comparatively recent times.

RECENT HISTORY

Naturopathy was in effect rediscovered in the 19th century, through the radical efforts of those who found the prevailing medical practices unacceptable. Medical thinking had not progressed much further than its first step from the Middle Ages: scholarly physicians who regarded the work of surgeons as a messy admission of failure and apothecaries, who carried out a dispensing role, akin to much of today's general practice. Their remedies however, were brutal – bleeding and blistering, vomiting and purging, potions of deadly elements of a 'heroic' kind.

The reformers who were not medically trained, are regarded as some of naturopathy's outstanding lay contributors. Often they were unconventionally religious or naturalist in outlook. Vincent Priessnitz (1799–1852), a farmer from Silesia in eastern Europe, promoted nutritional and hydrotherapies based on his methods of caring for his farm animals, and the importance of environment, in particular air and light, was emphasized by Arnold Rikli (1823–1906) at his lakeside centre in Slovenia.

Not only did the new naturopathic practitioners propose alternative treatments for ill-health, they were also acutely critical of accepted views of its causation. While this could make for a distinctly uncomfortable life for those with medical colleagues, at the same time less resistant doctors felt able to take on fresh ideas from unconventional practitioners.

What distinguished the naturopathic approach was its restating of the pure Hygienist principle that ill-health was unwise living, and the assertion that people could regain health with the minimum of doctoring. So prevalent was the view that life's imperfections had to be medically corrected that the new practitioners were promptly derided as 'ungodly' or 'unscientific'. Yet within a few years eminent doctors such as Dr Osler (quoted here) were willing to admit:

> The change is great. This new treatment relies very greatly on the so-called natural methods, diet and exercise, bathing and massage;

in other words, giving the natural forces their fullest scope by easy and thorough nutrition, increased circulation and removal of obstructions to the eliminative systems.

Naturopathic treatment for typhoid, a scourge of those times, was given by Dr Osler as an example:

> The patient is bathed and nursed and carefully tended but rarely given medicine. In comparison with other treatments, it was perfectly certain that the new practitioners lost no more of their patients than other doctors. There was but one conclusion: that most drugs had no effect whatsoever on the diseases for which they were administered.

THE RISE OF 'SCIENTIFIC' MEDICINE AND BIOMEDICINE

The notion that health's imperfections were caused by the agency of entities – formerly by demons and latterly by micro-organisms – is perhaps a carry-over from the Dark Ages. Unfortunately, just when naturopathy might have succeeded in influencing the rationale for treating symptoms, a development took place which was to dictate the entire course of medical practice: the fusion of medical education with the introduction of pharmacology provided by large industrial manufacturers. By the beginning of the 20th century the decision to have an exclusively 'science-based', interventionist medicine, to the exclusion of other approaches, was confirmed. To ensure that this would be successful, generous funding for medical education was provided by the industrialists themselves. Not only was non-drug-based health care stigmatized as quackery, but it was also not able to compete educationally or financially for practitioners.

Biomedicine

With the 20th century well under way, modern health care had become biomedicine, a drug therapy administered by practitioners who might examine their patients, but need not necessarily know much about their lives. It simplified the consultation process; any doctor could treat a patient as long as the appropriate drug was available. This was indeed an improvement on the sordid and lengthy deliberations of medieval medicine, if only from the position of the doctor. And for some time it gave the appearance of unqualified success – fewer people suffered and died from the diseases of former times.

However, in the midst of the self-congratulation and the promise of even greater achievement, medical observers known as epidemiologists were compiling reports of something of which the busy doctors were becoming increasingly aware: that the incidence of previously uncommon conditions such as cancers was rising; that more people were dying from diseases of the cardiovascular system; that conditions were emerging which seemed resistant even to the most favoured drug, the antibiotic. Furthermore, populations who were apparently well provided for were beginning to exhibit premature degeneration.

By the mid 1960s the world's cultures were showing signs of convergence. To a new Western generation, sufficiently detached from colonialism, Oriental influences, antique and exotic, attracted closer attention. India welcomed the world to its centres of spirit and culture. It became possible to visit China. The philosophies of indigenous peoples, as diverse as the North American Indians and Australian Aborigines were found to resonate with Hygieia's principles. Suddenly modern medicine appeared to be a superficial, if necessary, aspect of the total requirement for health care.

But having assumed the central role, biomedicine was reluctant to share the responsibility. A relationship of co-operation with the pharmaceutical industry had led to a form of drug dependence. Not only did major companies supply the medicines which doctors prescribed, they were the source of funding for treatment programmes for newer drugs.

THE 'FRINGE'

Pioneers of Naturopathy

Naturopathy was consigned to relatively small private projects, by lakesides or on mountain tops, from which much of the stereotypical views of its practice are derived. Yet the Hygienically inspired movement continued to develop, albeit gradually and rather exclusively, especially in the USA. There, some conventional doctors, influenced by contact with immigrant practitioners, took up naturopathy. Training schools were established, with the result that many Europeans went to the USA to be trained and returned home to reintroduce naturopathy to Europe.

James Thomson and Stanley Lief share the distinction of having brought naturopathy to prominence in the UK at the turn of this century. Both established residential clinics, Thomson in Scotland and Lief in southern England. From these two centres, a new generation of practitioners emerged, who took naturopathy further afield, as far away as Australia and New Zealand.

Dr Gordon Latto's work has also been a major influence in raising consciousness among medical doctors. Having trained simultaneously in Britain and naturopathically oriented Germany, Dr Latto has maintained a naturopathic practice near London for sixty years.

The Impact of the 'Fringe'

Perhaps the 19th-century naturopathic reformers were reincarnated Oriental or indigenous people before their time.

Those who took up the mantle in the 20th century were at least acknowledged, albeit disparagingly, by the mainstream as 'fringe practitioners'. The fringe included some therapies which had maintained a growing influence throughout plus the Oriental approaches which were Hygienic, in that they stressed lifestyle treatment.

The impact of the 'fringe' on orthodoxy was mixed: sometimes acceptable where it fell into the fashionable aspects of medicine, but often rejected as irreligious, especially where the emphasis was placed on the inner resources of the patient. Conventional criticism was gentler than previously but the philosophical divide remained: getting people to feel better about themselves was not as scientific as *making* them better.

The increased circulation of ideas amongst professionals eventually filtered down to patients, and there was a rising concern about the safety of biomedical treatments. Sometimes individuals would report sudden almost allergic reactions to drugs to which they thought they had become accustomed; others reported the sudden onset of unrecognizable symptoms from longer-term drug therapy. This gave birth to a novel diagnosis: iatrogenesis – becoming more unwell as a direct result of treatment.

As had happened previously, some conventional practitioners began openly to question their procedures and adopt a more naturopathic position. Naturopathic training schools flourished and the 'fringe' seemed to have the potential to become a medical alternative. A full philosophical circle had turned within a century and it looked as if it could be in the form of an upward spiral.

THE PRESENT DAY

The 1990s have ushered in a more politically correct concept of complementary medicine. The new definition still retains biomedicine in its central Asclepian position, but is integrated with complementary therapies which are founded on Hygieia's principles. At present, this is very much at the concept stage but the signs are encouraging. An example of this at a professional level was the creation of the post of Professor of Complementary Medicine at a leading UK university in 1992. Only a few years ago doctors were debarred from even referring a patient to a non-conventional practitioner.

Clinically, recent events have indicated a need for awareness similar to that of Priessnitz, for example, in that the mistreatment of domestic farm animals has unavoidable consequences for the fate of human life. Less predictably, who could have foreseen that Rikli's belief in the importance of pure air and light, ridiculed as an obsession in his day, would become today's most pressing environmental concern?

Unquestionably, the healing of the split between the two original Greek traditions is in the best interests of all. While the initiative would still appear to be with biomedicine, responsibility for maintaining momentum is an obligation shared equally between health-care consumers and naturopathic professionals.

Naturopathy is critical about institutionalized conventional medicine while acknowledging skilful medical practice. It does not support the view that so called 'natural therapies' are always more desirable than the appropriate use of pharmaceuticals or surgery. Natural therapy is not exclusively concerned with working with nature, any more than a surgeon can be successful without relying on natural wound healing. Also, certain developmental and genetic disorders, complex chronic conditions and illnesses which are extremely painful are clearly outwith the general application of naturopathy.

Strict adherence to natural therapy would in fact mean no therapy at all. However, modern medical culture has tended to swing our attitudes towards the opposite extreme – the view that we can ignore our fundamental bio-logicality, that pain is insignificant and should be eliminated without addressing its cause, and that the length of an individual's life should be extended indefinitely, without regard for quality.

It is doubtful whether today's more informed population will become the passive patients of former times. This new situation favours naturopathy's integration into 21st-century health care.

PSYCHO-NEURO-ENDOCRINO-IMMUNOLOGY (PNEI)

This conventional expression is as near as orthodox medicine has reached in approaching the concept of naturopathy. Loosely translated it suggests: 'Our thoughts and feelings are intimately connected to the workings and maintenance of our body.' It is not yet widely practised but is at the research forefront of an emerging medical view, which is currently attracting different clinicians who have gone so far in to their specialization as to confront its limitations. In particular, it is beginning to enlighten the materialistic logic of immunity, with the possibility of revolutionizing ways in which people experiencing everyday disorders and with potentially devastating conditions such as cancer and heart disease are treated.

PNEI is tentatively stating what generations of naturopathic practice and many individuals' intuitive experience bears out: that even where the provocation for disease exists externally, the susceptibility of a person to succumb to disease seems to depend on an inner, personal profile. This has to be suggested delicately because it is not intended to shift the blame for illness on to the patient. Rather, it is an empowerment, a shift from helplessness and an opportunity to discover meaning in the condition of being unwell, which even the most sophisticated medical treatments have not begun to address.

This development fortunately comes at a time when the wisdom of orthodoxy's principal contributions, the widespread use of antibiotics and childhood vaccination are under current review. Although both medicines make an initial impact on disease processes, they belong to the most denying, alienating forms of treatment. New research clearly indicates that antibiosis at best merely postpones the manifestation of symptoms and occasionally, in the case of certain vaccinations, converts disorders into more complicated conditions. Naturopathy has consistently been able to draw attention to people's extreme reactions to this form of treatment, since it has caused many people to seek naturopathic help. The new research has tended to confirm the undesirable effects of denying symptoms on the wider population.

Being 'immune' is not a product of a sterile environment. It has ultimately to do with *adaptability*, the main reason why populations survived before medical interventions. Naturopathy asserts that, in spite of the dramatically polluted and over-populated world it inhabits, the human body still possesses the inner mechanical, chemical and cerebral resources to ensure its healthy survival.

The following are areas in which PNEI research and naturopathic treatment concur:

- Follow your appetite. *Eat well* (the ingredients in raw foods are important enough to be called 'protective') or *not at all* (short fasting releases more healing hormones).
- *Move* as much of the body as possible (it is in partnership with your heart and circulation is all) but also *rest* whenever you are tired (night sleeping needs to be complemented).
- Have a *positive* attitude or at least be *receptive to healing* (cleansing white blood cells increase in number).
- Have a *reason* to get well and to be well (research shows that survivors have more than courage).

If naturopathic treatment is so straightforward and effective, it is sometimes asked, why is it not used universally? One answer is that it is probably practised more than is formally recognized, but not with full confidence.

Spontaneous self-care is usually naturopathic in principle but the pressure to have one's condition medicalized is great. It is also natural to feel the need to be in the care of another person when one is unwell and exclusively naturopathic practitioners are rare. However, more and more conventional medical practice is becoming 'ecological' and naturopathic tendencies are seen to be emerging with new generations of medical practitioners. Surgeons, in particular, would accept that naturopathic care is an appropriate preparation for an operation.

Some patients seek naturopathic help after disappointment with conventional care but the majority are keen to maintain their health by combining the best of both biomedicine and naturopathy. It is not always possible to follow an exclusively 'natural' course of treatment since patients may be dependent on long-term medication or have been subject to disrupting surgery.

Normally, benefits of treatment are seen over a period of time, especially if a condition has been slowly building up. Practitioners work on the basis of one month in treatment to address each past year of disorder.

Naturopaths are accustomed to many patients 'signing-off' from treatment sessions without formal acknowledgement. This can be disconcerting in the early days of practice but the nature of treatment encourages independence in the patient. The more successful the consultation, the more likely the patient is to take disorder in their stride and want to get on with a revitalized life. When a patient reappears much later at the practice, enquiries about a former condition are invariably met with 'Oh, yes, that just cleared up.'

2

The Principles of Naturopathy

*[Conventional] medical science and services are misdirected, and
society's investment in health is not well used, because they rest
on an erroneous assumption about the basis of human health.
This approach has led to indifference to the external influences
and personal behaviour which are the predominant determinants
of health.*

*Thomas McKeown, former Professor of Social Medicine at the
University of Birmingham, England*

NATUROPATHY IS A PHILOSOPHY which provides a health-care
approach but offers much more than merely an alternative
medical system. It encompasses a view of life, a purpose in
human health and suffering and a model for living a full life.

It strongly affirms the benevolence of life and recommends
simple lifestyle measures to meet the reality of health problems.
It is rational, yet it takes into account an individual's idio-
syncrasies. It is also original and truly therapeutic, in that its
guiding principles for a healthy life are identical to the treatment
for ill-health, the difference being only in emphasis.

HEALTH IS DETERMINED BY NUTRITION

Naturopathy upholds that the single most important determinant
of health is nutrition. In gardening, in caring for domestic
animals and in rearing farm livestock, it is generally accepted
that a failure to thrive or reproductive difficulties are primarily a
problem of faulty nutrition. In humans, beyond early infant

feeding, we observe that as life expands, nutritional concerns tend to diminish until a state of omniverousness is attained.

Having the capacity to ingest almost anything, however, is not the same as having the ability to be nourished at random. Naturopaths recognize that for optimum functioning other creatures appear to choose from sources which can be best utilized by their digestive systems. In this respect, our basic nutritional requirements would be resourced directly from plants, supplemented by concentrated foods which provide energy and repair.

HEALTH IS MOVEMENT

Naturopathy stresses the importance of movement and posture. The human body is a true marvel, having the potential to equal, and on many levels excel, the physical capabilities of all other creatures. This is almost entirely due to our unique uprightness. Evolution has ensured that by simply enjoying the use of our bodies as they are designed, we retain our uniqueness and derive much satisfaction from life. Conversely, our flexibility, strength, co-ordination and ultimately our prized poise, are forfeited if we do not use them.

The freely moving body also contributes to organic health, since external movement causes inner massage-like effects which help maintain the organs of the body by improving circulation. Movement also dissipates excessive nervous tension, which restores balance to the neurological workings of the body. Naturopathy uses massage to help to improve posture and to encourage the body's own internal rhythmic movements which assist the functioning of the internal organs.

HEALTH IS PSYCHO-PHYSIOLOGICAL

According to naturopathy, the distinction between body and mind is artificial and without meaning for an individual. The concept of separateness is only useful for the analysis of apparently different levels of activity within us, and in many ways is disrespectful to a person. Times of distress can be polarizing, however, and we have become accustomed to directing body symptoms to physicians, leaving feelings and emotions exclusively to psychiatric medicine. Naturopathy accepts this situation in order to deliver a therapeutic paradox. In order to enter into the cycle of psycho-physiological being, the more 'physical' the symptom, the more psychologically accented is the treatment; where symptoms are emotionally centred, physical treatments are recommended. The effect of this is to loosen up the intensity of symptoms and mobilize the patient's available energy for healing.

ONE HEALTH, ONE DISEASE

Perhaps this is the central principle of naturopathy. This proposes that if, as most people would accept, there is only one 'health', it is not unreasonable to accept only one disease, namely the absence of health, rather than a catalogue of pathological entities.

Initially, this might sound preposterous, given the myriad diagnosed conditions to be found in the volumes of the *International Classification of Diseases* (ICD) and the many specialized professions operating within mainstream medicine. It becomes clear, however, from observation of medical practice that the labelling of illness is primarily for the benefit of the profession; it is not designed to give insight to the patient. A typical example of this is when a patient complains of many painful and inflamed joints. A biomedical doctor will diagnose polyarticular arthritis, which is literally translated as 'hot joints everywhere'! This expression might usefully define the extent of the condition for the doctor, or eliminate other possibilities; but for the non-Latin speaking patient, however, a diagnosis in alien textbook terminology can confirm feelings of disintegration at a time when reassurance and support may be most needed instead.

This process of creating disease entities, which has always been a feature of psychiatric medicine, is a sophistication of infantile fears. Here, diagnosis can be elevated to the level of treatment in itself, for the lack of any other options. It is perhaps an understandable human need to have a name for some emotional suffering, in that it may help relieve its burden. But a diagnostic process which alienates someone from what really exists as part of themselves at that time is of questionable value.

A currently fashionable contender for addition to the *ICD*, for example, is polymorph dysfunction disorder — literally 'dissatisfied with physical appearance' – which suggests that diagnosis has reached the point of disassociation.

Naturopathy's 'one health' emphasizes that it is more important for patients to develop their own vocabulary during illness. Rather than rejection, gentle identification with one's condition is recommended. Given that ill-health can make people fearful, this can sound a daunting prospect but it is made possible by a revolutionary attitude toward symptoms.

THE SYMPTOMS OF ILL-HEALTH ARE FRIENDLY

At this stage it becomes necessary to define two terms which are often confused: symptoms and signs. *Symptoms* are the subjective experiences of the sufferer, whereas *signs* are the observations of the practitioner. 'My headache makes me feel drained' is an example of a symptom, while 'The headache makes the patient look pale' is recorded as a sign.

Signs are measurable, quantifiable and comparable, and make up much of the statistical information which describes ill-health. Once the signs have been identified, orthodox treatments are usually directed towards eliminating symptoms, for example, anti-inflammatory medicine or surgical removal. According to naturopathy, this approach is questionably short-term but more importantly, denies the patient the opportunity of insight into his or her condition.

Although symptoms are sometimes frightening and usually disturbing, naturopaths suggest that they are in fact expressions of intuition. Although it is understandable to feel resentful towards distress, everyday experience suggests that a 'friendly' message is usually contained within the simplest experience of pain. To resent this to the point of eliminating symptoms without understanding them, is merely to distort and postpone pain.

Naturopaths compare symptoms to fragments of upsetting dreams, which represent actions or events of which we have become unconscious. Although they are initially unrecognizable, an identification with symptoms is a logical stage in naturopathic treatment if illness is to have any purpose.

For example, few people will have escaped the experience of swollen glands, which is the temporary inflammation and enlargement of the lymphatic nodes found under the arm or in the groin or throat. Rather than being life-threatening, hyperactivity of these structures is very life-preserving, being a normal response to an unacknowledged period of physical or emotional stress. Without this response, the system would be unable to eliminate potentially poisoning wastes quickly.

Yet the orthodox treatment for this complaint is antibiotic medicine, which aims to reduce the activity of the nodes, because they apparently make the sufferer uncomfortable. The patient's perception may be further distorted by the implication that an entity is attacking the nodes. Naturopathy finds this bizarre. Not only is this treatment physically illogical but it detaches the patient from the realization that the system has been overworked and is showing the strain. It is not an exaggeration to suggest that the treatment itself constitutes a stressful event. Naturopathic treatment, using diet and hydrotherapy, helps manage the discomfort from the nodes without interfering with their functioning.

ACUTE CONDITIONS ARE UNAVOIDABLE

Acute illness is regarded as transient, self-limiting and common. In fact it is so common that we might suppose either that human beings are morbid creatures who become progressively ill until they die or perhaps that common conditions might wrongly be interpreted as illnesses. A naturopathic analysis of health suggests that the latter may be the case.

Acute conditions are invariably manifestations of the eliminative organs, suggesting that they are effectively extensions of normal activity. The skin is a particularly prominent player in acute disorders, for example:

- eczema – an inflamed condition which can be considered as an exaggerated 'blushing'
- Raynaud's syndrome – poor circulation in the extremities, a sign of withdrawal
- psoriasis – a dry, scaly condition, exaggerating the skin's defensiveness

To treat these conditions with suppressive medicine is to interfere with the normal mechanisms of the skin.

Naturopaths also observe that the many digestive conditions, which account for the majority of 'over the counter' prescriptions, appear to be associated with nervous disorder. When the parasympathetic nervous system is dominating, through drawn-out distress, it becomes impossible for the normally well co-ordinated process of digestion and elimination to occur. Upper digestion is incomplete, the linings of organs can become irritated, and eliminative functioning is erratic. It is of no therapeutic advantage to give each of these conditions a separate diagnostic term if they derive from a single neurological agency. Perhaps this is why it is becoming increasingly likely that digestive problems are ascribed to the syndrome of 'stress'.

A feature of common conditions is that they inconveniently interrupt our lives, causing either adaptation or complete cessation of activities. Another common finding is that people often feel particularly energetic prior to 'going down' with illness. Though it is not always consciously appreciated, someone may say that they feel so much better not just after being ill but *from* being ill, for example, they may feel 'much clearer' or 'stronger'.

CHRONIC CONDITIONS ARISE FROM THE MISMANAGEMENT OF ACUTE ILLNESSES

Disorders are usually defined as 'chronic' when severe degenerative processes such as osteoarthritis or bronchitis become established. Without being able to amass the type of conclusive evidence favoured in orthodox medicine, on the basis of observation and increasing recognition of iatrogenic (medically induced) complications, naturopaths contend that much chronicity is the outcome of the mistaken treatment of acute illness.

We are inclined to associate degeneration with images of 'wear and tear' on the body, but the population does not appear to wear out consistently enough to make this a generalization. To further confuse the situation, there are some who run the risk of a serious illness – by heavy smoking, for example – but do not develop it. Also, some who consistently carry heavy loads are not especially prone to degeneration of the spine, but display the quite the opposite condition.

Heart disease, which accounts for the greatest premature mortality in Western societies, is often thought to 'strike down' victims. Indeed, there are occasions when damaging heart conditions do not appear to be preceded by circulatory warnings, but often there are neurological mishaps or digestive irregularities. While they may not be connected within the specialist approach of conventional care, minor symptoms are not without significance in the one-health image of naturopathy.

ILLNESS BEGINS THE CURE

Even taking into account the pharmacological advances of recent times, the increased incidence of non-infectious illness suggests that an aggressive search for the cure of individual conditions has not been successful. Moreover, in the attempt to destroy the microbial aspects of illness, new, resistant superstrains of microbes have emerged.

In contrast, naturopathy defines a cure of embracing qualities, using ways of treatment which will extend life and improve its quality during ageing. To achieve this, disassociation, denial or phobia towards the manifestation of illness is unhelpful. Radically, naturopathy invites us to include the discomfort, upheaval and disorientation of illness as a necessary part of health. We are encouraged to accept that the demands we ourselves make upon our life, as well as those imposed by other factors, will naturally require periods of physical reorganization and biological adjustment.

THE CURE IS REST

We must have water, food and human contact in some form, but rest is also a fundamental need. Failure to rest sufficiently and appropriately often explains the escalation and intensity of symptoms.

The most obvious cue for rest is when appetite disappears. Since the digestion and processing of food takes a considerable amount of the body's energy it is a clear that missing a meal or two provides a useful rest period from physical or emotional strain. This indication is often accompanied by a sore throat or nausea, which makes the passage of food quite distressing, but if we follow the idea that it is necessary to eat to keep up our strength, we might still feel compelled to try. Ironically, the sludgy food which it is just possible to consume under these circumstances is the kind which is guaranteed to cause the digestion most work. Missing the occasional meal is hardly dangerous especially for people in well-fed, affluent societies who are estimated to have up to one month's energy stored within their liver.

Sleep may not be altogether restful but we get more rest by retiring early, not only before midnight but as soon as possible after 5pm. This is because our system begins its deeply regenerative work from this time onwards and we make more energy available by being unconscious. The daytime 'nap' is often not possible but the idea can be simply modified to a short break, with legs well elevated and back muscles relaxed. Naturopaths consider that treatments will not bring long-lasting benefits if they are not accompanied by increased rest.

NATUROPATHY AFFIRMS REALITY

The hope that we can always be well or that we can rely on scientific discoveries to eradicate all illnesses is an illusion that is increasingly being rejected, even by conventional medicine. After many decades of experimentation and research, it is clear that the majority of problems presented to practitioners are associated with a way of living rather than by assaults from life itself. This is true whether the disorder is attributed to pathological entities preying on innocent human life or portrayed in negative images of the body, as in, 'a *bad* back'. It is unfortunate that for many people this view becomes a consideration only after they have been disappointed by major medical or surgical intervention.

The principles of naturopathy may at first seem either naive or too radical for those who have previously relied exclusively on the biomedical system. The belief that fluctuations in well-being are unconnected with our behaviour or emotional environment is fostered from an early age in Western societies. For others, naturopathy may sound refreshingly familiar, and may confirm ideas they already possess.

Naturopaths acknowledge that not every medically diagnosed condition will respond predictably to naturopathy. Yet even in extreme conditions, where quality of life is paramount, naturopathic care still offers a most positive, person-affirming focus. The flexibility of its approach invites its application from the onset of symptoms, alongside any other treatments which are deemed necessary, and as a valuable aspect of convalescence and recovery.

3

Naturopathy in Practice

Healing is more than merely taking on a greater responsibility for my own well-being. It's an entirely new way of looking at health, illness and medicine. In particular, I've realized two things: that all illness represents an opportunity to learn about ourselves and the world we inhabit and create, and that chronic illness in particular challenges us to ask if it is possible to be successfully ill.

Tim Brookes, author - reflecting on his life
as an asthmatic

WHILE URGING US to develop a philosophical perspective on health, naturopathy also offers practical help in maintaining well-being. This is very important because although reactions to accidents and other major life interruptions, especially loss, can have a great impact on health, naturopaths often record that symptoms of illness are just as likely to arise from the ways we live our daily lives.

With the constant pressure and distractions of existence, it is perhaps easy to forget that our everyday routines are almost unconscious. It is important, therefore, to realize that much of what of our life is founded upon has been deliberately chosen. By reminding us of our basic self-direction, naturopathy is able to influence us at a fundamental level. Habits and responses are, of course, notoriously difficult to alter or even adapt. Naturopathy succeeds by explaining the attractive options: a more conscious life, with confidence in our own powers, and an increased understanding of the process of self-healing.

26

NUTRITION

While there appears to be a general consensus amongst health professionals on the need for a healthy diet, nutrition concerns much more than the food on our plate. With the exception of dental care and the dietary management of metabolic disorders, the study of nutrition has not been a major feature of the orthodox understanding of illness. There has until very recently been a reluctance to infringe on our personal freedom to choose exactly what we include in our diet. For the naturopath, the daily habits that most influence our health are connected with the way we are nourished.

Irrefutable evidence of the primary importance of nutrition was confirmed by epidemiological studies conducted by Professor Thomas McKeown and published in 1980. Epidemiology involves examining evidence from large populations, rather than isolated cases, to establish trends or explanations of illness, which makes Professor McKeown's findings all the more compelling. Reviewing medical statistics in the UK from 1900 to 1970, he clearly showed that the influence of nutrition exceeded that of any other health measure, including medical intervention. That this seemed true even in the case of infectious disease was an unexpected confirmation of the naturopathic view from within conventional medicine. It is not surprising that, given McKeown's conclusion that medical practice could profitably be pruned back to consist of merely the dentist, the accident surgeon and, with a few reservations, the obstetrician, conventional medicine did not embrace his findings.

Other researchers, such as Weston Price, a dentist who travelled world-wide in the 1920s, observed that indigenous peoples suffered illnesses previously rare when their nutritious diets were displaced by the processed foods eaten by Westerner traders. Apart from the physical effects which he was able to record, Price heard of psychological disorders, including suicide – hitherto unknown in some communities.

Obvious as these observations may seem, it has taken a dramatic rise in the 20th-century 'lifestyle' illnesses all around the world for the focus within mainstream medicine on the implications of diet on health to develop.

The difficulty in translating these findings into action for the public at large is that while we appear to have free choice in what we eat, in reality our choices are already conditioned by strong external influences. The most powerful among these is that we obtain our food from the food manufacturing industry and not, as in the past, the growers, hand in hand with nature. For the manufacturers to maintain their dominance they have to process food, which they do by preserving, eg by adding salt, and occasionally, by disassembling it, as is done to wheat and sugar cane.

Salt is an 'anti-nutrient', in that consumption results in a loss of valuable minerals from the body. This has a 'pickling' effect, where the softer tissues of the body are hardened, and the firm tissues are softened. Excessive intakes of salt, which may occur even from low doses over long periods, are now believed to play a major role in degenerative conditions of the heart, lungs and bones.

Refined carbohydrate obtained from wheat and sugar has been clearly shown to initiate a number of disorders, from tooth decay to other less visible but serious conditions. Refining foods inevitably leads to overconsumption, undoubtedly a commercial triumph, but that gives rise to obesity, which is considered to be a greater threat to health than undernutrition.

Confusingly for the general public, 'expert' advice about food can also be subject to fashion, even within respectable scientific circles. Dietary recommendations often reflect ideals which are either impractical or unattainable. Over sixty years ago, when many people were so poor as to be subsisting on a one-course main meal of the day, the following was promoted as the ideal menu:

- first course: *hors d'oeuvres* – colourful, spicy foods to stimulate the appetite
- second course: soup – to warm the mouth and stomach
- third course: fish – to extend the time of the meal
- main course: meat, gravy, vegetables – to produce satiety
- sweet: to extend satiety
- cheese: to remove the after-taste of the meal, with biscuits to scrub and clean the tongue
- coffee: to stimulate a tiring digestion
- cigarette: to fumigate the mouth and offset sleepiness

Contemporary diners are sometimes presented with specific advice, an example being the butter/margarine controversy. Here, fat within butter is linked to deposits found on our blood vessels, which raises pressure and restricts circulation, while margarine apparently does not. Whatever the technical evidence of this might be, margarine is a highly refined vegetable product which is sold on the nutritional value of the whole plant, from which it is derived. Admittedly, butter is only part of whole milk but it has not been subject to the processing of margarine, and will give a clear indication of its freshness.

LEARNING FROM BABIES

An individual's diet may have emotional connotations – eg 'man's food' – or an attachment to family customs or values. Food can also assume a psychological significance, becoming a replacement for unsatisfied needs or compensation for complex feelings of emptiness. Naturopathy appreciates that recommending one type of diet for all people is an oversimplification and uses a rather obvious model for nutrition, to which every human being can relate: our experience as babies.

Observation of babies reveals three useful points: first, babies consume fresh food; secondly, although toothless, babies 'chew' well before swallowing; and thirdly, babies feed contentedly when they are comfortable and refrain when they are not.

What to Eat: Fresh as Possible

A healthy mother's breast milk is designed to be the most perfect human food. It contains the perfect balance of nutrients and protective agents, which justifies the saying of Hippocrates that 'food should be our medicine and medicine our food'; its temperature is ideal; it is microbiologically clean; above all, although it might be warm, it is unprocessed.

A cursory glance inside a well-stocked supermarket reveals that while formerly foods were bought for their freshness, technology and packaging have allowed processed foods to dominate the shopping basket. Food companies spend far more on promoting processed foods than fresh ones because of their increased profitability. Fresh foods are profiled as interesting but inconvenient, compared to ready-prepared, long-lasting alternatives. Perhaps too, in a bizarre sense, the instant availability of processed foods is like an ever-ready breast!

Dr M O Bircher-Benner, a Swiss doctor-nutritionist showed

that eating fresh foods, especially at the beginning of meals, maximized vitamin and mineral absorption. Japanese food researcher Professor Katsuyne and his wife experimented by adopting a daily diet containing only the number of calories given in labour camps but in the form of raw foods. They remained well for three months then changed to the same calories in processed foods. Within one month, they became so unwell they had to abandon the experiment.

Eat food for its freshness, not calories. Eat raw when possible and at the start of a meal.

How to Eat: Chewing and Breathing

Although breast milk is fluid, it is eliminated from babies as a solid. As if in recognition of this, babies do not swallow their milk as a drink but circulate it around the mouth in a primitive jawing. Babies also appear to breathe well while feeding. If the nasal passages are blocked and they feed for extended periods and breathe through the mouth, indigestion occurs.

An adult's mouth contains three types of teeth for different actions: canines for tearing, incisors for chopping and molars for grinding. The jaws not only open and close when chewing but also move from side to side. This also gives our food a chance to be mixed with juices released from glands within the mouth, which begin the process of digestion. Using our whole mouth results in a solid food being liquefied before being swallowed.

Food enters our blood combined with oxygen in a process known as metabolism. Without effective breathing, therefore, even the best food and most efficient digestion will not help. It is not necessary for adults to breathe during meals in exactly the same way that feeding babies breathe; however, simple deep-breathing exercises performed daily will help to maximize nutritional intake.

Breathing through the mouth often happens inadvertently, and produces an even more complicated indigestion problem than that experienced by a baby. For the adult, indigestion is usually sited in the large intestine, where it manifests as gas or, if it is retained, causes an undesirable stretching of the colon wall.

Take time to enjoy the sensation of eating; speak after swallowing. Increase exercise rather than food to get more energy.

When to Eat: Be Comfortable as Well as Hungry

Food is consumed not only for sustenance but also when we feel
bored or frustrated, and often as a response to being alarmed or
agitated. The latter, known as 'comfort eating', is reminiscent of
our needs in infancy. The type of foods which adults tend to
choose for comfort – starchy and sweet – are certainly similar to
infant foods but they do not compare as nutrition.

However, eating when confronted by a threat may be a useful,
stress-relieving activity, if gorilla behaviour is anything to go by.
These powerful, supremely confident creatures, when encountering stress-provoking conditions do not instantly beat their chests
as is commonly supposed. Rather, they reach for their favourite
plants and begin eating in a particularly nonchalant way, as if to
minimize the threat. This certainly conserves energy in comparison with an unnecessary over-reaction, but the behaviour is
also interesting in a subtle sense. Although it is apparently eating,
the gorilla merely chews the leaves and then spits them out.

Restricting our food intake totally or partially, as a fast when
we feel unwell, may have benefits we are only just beginning to
be able to measure. It would seem logical that if we have no
appetite, with a swollen throat or bowel upset, we will feel dis-
inclined to eat much. Yet we are brought up to believe that
eating gives immediate strength and without food we would not
have the energy to recover from illness. In fact research by
conventional doctors from the University of Australia would
seem to confirm that the opposite is true. The strength which is
gained from fasting is not muscular but hormonal, and having
conducted experiments on volunteers, Professor Ray Kearney
and Dr Gavin Greenock concluded that our body's natural anti-
inflammatory response, via the hormones known as corticosteroids, is increased when food is restricted.

The conclusions drawn from this research suggest that
concentrated foods are best consumed within any one six-hour
period of the day, with only raw foods eaten in the remaining
period. The authors recommend this for the typical inflammation
of acute illness, as well as for degenerative conditions such as
cancer.

Extensive clinical studies of fasting in Sweden show that
human beings do not require food in the way that, for example, a
motor vehicle requires fuel. The famous Stockholm marches, led

by Dr Lennart Edren, illustrated this. Nineteen men walked from Gothenburg to Stockholm, a distance of over 325 miles, in ten days, while on a total fast. Moreover, their protein and blood sugar levels were shown to be normal throughout the fasting period. In fact, a number of the men felt so much stronger on reaching Stockholm than they had before the march, that they immediately turned round and walked back to Gothenburg!

If you are uneasy, in pain or unwell, drink easy-to-digest raw food juices; restrict concentrated 'energy' foods, which may be debilitating.

POSTURE AND MOVEMENT

The human body has evolved to give us the maximum possible strength, flexibility and co-ordination. To achieve this we have 'borrowed' design features from all other creatures so that although we can be outrun, outclimbed or outswum, no other animal can compete with us in a 'triathalon'.

In the face of the many mechanical disorders which abound – low back pain, prolapsed organs and eye strain to name but a few – it is sometimes believed that we have attained our supreme posture at a high price. Naturopathy suggests that problems of posture and movement are more often a reflection of underuse or abuse rather than precarious design. For example, carrying heavy loads certainly seems to invite back strain, yet Kenyan women have demonstrated that they are able to carry up to 20 per cent of their own body weight before any increase in back tension is recorded. That this is achieved by carrying the load on top of their head illustrates two points: first, that for the average person pain may be indicating that back muscles are being used wrongly; and secondly, that perhaps our arms are not especially suited to carrying.

The skeleton is extremely robust, our leg bones being as strong as teak. The joints which enable us to move our arms and legs freely are so well constructed that it is estimated that they could last 150 years' regular use. The most dreaded disease of the bone is not suffering a multiple fracture from use, however, but softening of our bones, osteoporosis, which is a result of underuse. There may be hormonal factors which contribute towards bones becoming porous in later life; however, the formation of the sturdy, compact layer of a bone is ensured by continually stressing the skeleton from an active life, rather than sparing it. Similarly, the disfiguring, incapacitating swelling of our joints known as arthritis, is not associated with overuse but with insufficient movement.

Our muscles belong to one co-ordinated system. Although they are individually named to identify their direction of movement, almost all muscles take part in every action. Reaching out with our arms increases the muscle tone in our backs; sitting down causes our necks to become tighter; standing on one leg requires complete muscular control. All this becomes quite apparent when only one muscle is injured – even the simplest action feels restricted.

Muscles also perform other vital functions. It is their movements, finding resistance against the skin, which help propel the blood back towards the heart. Muscles also absorb impact, both physically and emotionally – they literally help us 'bounce' back. Moreover, it is through our muscles and the postures they create, especially those of the face, that we communicate our strongest feelings. As babies, our physical independence begins when our muscles are able to hold our bones upright. The arrangement whereby the spine assumes a central position not only allows for liberating movements but also enables the organs of the body to work efficiently.

Strain

When being upright becomes tiring most animals simply lie down. Human beings have become accustomed to sitting, which in effect means sitting on the tail of the spine. This is actually not restful, as anyone who is suffering from back ache will testify. Especially over extended periods, sitting down is really partially collapsing, and introduces other forms of serious pressure to the body. This may be manifested in increased tension of the neck and lower back – 'slipped disc'; restricted breathing from collapsed chest – 'asthma'; the abdominal contents become unsupported and prolapse – 'haemorrhoids'; blood circulation is depressed and venous return, from the legs in particular, is impeded – 'varicose veins'.

Athletes, dancers and musicians learn the importance of posture in efficient performance but it took a Tasmanian actor, Frederick Mathias Alexander to demonstrate how vital posture is

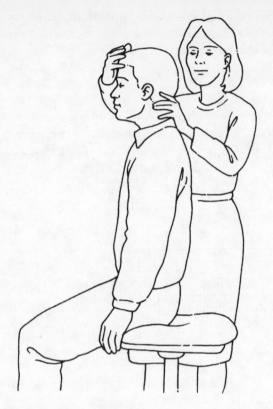

*Figure 2   The Alexander Technique: the teacher gently alters your position
minutely in order to release tension*

to everyday life. His discovery, that neck tension was interfering
with his acting, led to the development of the Alexander
Technique (AT). Acknowledging that we are destined to live in
a world of chairs, teachers of the technique use the motions
of sitting and standing to help explain how better posture can
be achieved. Teachers report improvements in back strain,
breathing and eyesight from using the technique.

Like naturopathy, AT emphasizes restoring normal functioning rather than removing obstructions. Its benefits come not
from eliminating body tension, but from loosening it so that it
becomes available for freer expression. It is stressed that AT is
not a fixed series of exercises but an exploration which encourages
a person to rediscover natural poise.

Imagine your body to be suspended from above rather than planted in the ground. Try to sit down slowly, without bumping onto the chair; stand up without moving your arms.

Yoga

Naturopaths also recommend, with qualification, the physical movements of yoga. The oneness of this philosophy interprets posture as defining both physical and mental attitude. Therefore in yoga practice, the positions which the body takes up influence not only bodily inflexibility but also underlying tension in thoughts and feelings. The qualification concerning yoga is that to be truly beneficial it needs to be studied initially with personal guidance. This is because, left to oneself, one's yoga practice can become tension-confirming or even suppressive.

There may be a tendency, for example, to adopt yoga postures which can be easily achieved rather than more challenging, complementary ones. Similarly, gentle abdominal breathing, which has a pacifying effect generally, may be inappropriate for someone who is required to meet specific situations with increasing assertiveness. An experienced practitioner, with a detached perspective, is able to help assess which aspect of yoga might be most appropriate.

Without the help of an experienced practitioner, the most beneficial yoga practice involves twisting, like slow 'wringing out', and positions which offer a degree of inversion – from simply raised legs to a shoulder-stand.

Massage

Naturopaths are skilled in the use of massage and manipulation to help restore and maintain posture. Massage is a very versatile therapy, which can be modified to meet the requirements of the individual. This is because the movements of massage are designed to follow the natural movements of the body. When expertly done, there is no massage stroke which the body does not recognize and no stroke which can interfere with its functioning. Smooth stroking and frictions stimulate the skin and help de-stress the nervous system; the muscles are invigorated by being squeezed and compressed; passive movement of joints helps reduce pressure and realign posture.

The lower back is given priority in massage, not only because it is easily strained but because the legs and abdomen are influenced by its tension. Massage of the lower back is especially indicated during pregnancy to relieve pressure and discourage lordosis – an accentuated inward curve of the spine.

Massage should be a pleasure which puts the 'treat' into treatment, and its benefits are not exclusive to professional therapy. Spontaneous but careful massage can be given within friendships and families, using gentle strokes, given within comfortable limits. Practitioners also recommend self-massage for fitness and relaxation.

Respond to aches and pains by trading massages, especially for the lower back, with a friend; regularly self-massage your abdomen and face. Do not delay seeking professional help for muscle and joint disorders.

EMOTION

Naturopathy describes emotion as a person's psychological movement. Although there are many expressions of emotion, naturopaths regard our emotional state as the 'bank balance' of our fundamental needs – to be nourished, to be safe, to belong and to contribute.

It is quite apparent that the evolutionary superiority conferred by human life does not guarantee, but possibly complicates, the fulfilment of these basic needs. Human beings display vulnerabilities beyond those observed in many other species. Naturopathy finds this quite understandable because having so many expectations to live up to, human life is inherently anxious.

Stress

Emotionality sometimes appears to represent an effort to remain poised between degrees of comfort and discomfort. Within the body this is characterized by the condition of that part of the nervous system known as the sympathetic and parasympathetic. These nerves constantly monitor our emotional requirements, giving cues to behaviours which are likely to fulfil them.

Unfortunately, these promptings may be in conflict with external constraints, usually in the form of others' needs. Unrelieved conflict leads to what is popularly termed 'stress'.

Stress becomes embodied as hypertensions: in the circulatory system (high blood pressure), in digestive spasm (irritable bowel) or in inflamed joints (arthritis). Naturopathy sees such examples of increased pressures as unacceptable compromises which invite more acceptable responses.

Emotions create the atmosphere of the body in the form of pressure. The most common source of increased pressure is conflict with others' emotional interests.

Anxiety

In the sports world it is observed that individuals can become 'injury-prone'. Naturopathy suggests that this type of vulnerability exists in everyday life in the form of predisposition – an underlying posture which emerges in the form of symptoms. Both states can be considered as an escape from intolerable conflict. For the athlete this may involve physical breakdown which clearly prevents participation; in everyday life, escape may take the form of symptoms which, although disabling, are not particularly life-threatening.

Clues as to why we might opt to produce symptoms rather than address our conflicts openly are available from studies conducted on injured sportspeople. For many athletes, their activity involves joining an extended family – the coach is a parent, the team is the family. Because of the emotional relationships this creates, in spite of the rewards of success and prestige, participation in sport is anxiety-provoking. It has been observed that sportspeople's injuries can be linked to a fear of failure, the avoidance of competition, redressing real or imagined grievances with team-mates, an attempt to frustrate dominant coaching and the maintenance of the illusion that, but for injury, greater success might have been achieved.

Similarly in everyday life, the pressure to conform, to meet others' expectations of us and to succeed can be just as demanding as in the competitive world of sport. Indeed, while the sportsperson has the option of graceful retirement from physical activity, our social pressures continue until the very end of life.

Naturopathy emphasizes that recognizing this may give a clue as to how best we might respond to symptoms.

Physical symptoms for which there are no apparent reasons may be considered as embodying emotional stress. Their source is likely to be social pressure.

Speaking Out

Naturopathy encourages the expression rather than suppression of symptoms. Through this it is possible to reach an understanding of one's condition instead of merely accepting a diagnostic label. Expression can take the form of a rise in body temperature, loss of appetite or the need to speak about something previously unspoken. Although wordiness can be part of an attempt to conceal emotion, being able to speak freely is also associated with emotional release, as in 'getting something off one's chest'.

Words are great conveyors of emotions, whether in the precise form they take, in their partially hidden allusions or in their simple poetry. Words can appear to 'escape' into conversations. The 'Freudian slip', where attention is drawn to a subject by inadvertent juxtaposition or by mispronouncing a word to make a more revealing statement than is consciously intended, is an experience known to most of us.

Therapeutically oriented conversations are often excluded from conventional consultations because of the practitioner's reluctance to 'stir things up'. Naturopathy considers this an unfounded fear. A conversation which facilitates speaking out can only use emotional material which is already conscious – it is already 'up'. Silence is not protective but isolating for the patient.

Similar concerns are raised about encouraging dependency. It would be cruel not to offer a walking stick to someone with a traumatized leg; while the stick is serving a purpose, it becomes a valid dependency. If, after the leg has recovered, a person feels that they cannot give up their stick, another issue arises, namely attachment, but this is not a direct problem of dependency. Without the stick, they would have been completely reliant on others.

In the same way, without being offered the opportunity to

speak, we can be denied another useful form of help. Practitioners should of course be alert to the possibility of attachment, which indicates a positive transition from primary trauma. If, however, a practitioner feels that they are encountering emotions which they find it difficult to work with, then there is always the option of referring the patient to a more suitable therapist. It is not in the patient's best interest to be told 'to pull oneself together' if falling apart is a part of being unwell.

For therapists whose work is dominated by the biomedical model of care, there is often a sense of failure if the patient becomes increasingly emotional. It may appear from the therapist's point of view as though the problem is becoming more chaotic, in spite of treatment. In the clinical scenario, this is seen in the offering of paper tissues to a patient who becomes tearful – the implicit message being 'dry up!' Naturopathic treatment, on the other hand, encompasses the facilitation of an emotional response. This is not simply an attempt to make an individual weep, but a recognition of the complexity of feeling which pervades illness.

Human language is the most sophisticated development of the body. It is not consistent with treating the rest of the body's heightened response to illness to regard our own words as irrelevant during this time. Conversations with carers are important during illness and should be encouraged. The aim of naturopathy is to work with the body's communications in all their guises, be these through the language of words or symptoms.

ALLOPATHY

Conventional medicines are designed to produce a counter-action, as is seen in their descriptions: *anti*biotic, *anti*-inflammatory, *anti*depressive. This approach, which is known as allopathy, is directed against the physical manifestation of symptoms. Its success is measured by how far symptoms can be exterminated. Given our present understanding of the biological processes of the body, naturopathy finds this a cynical method of treating symptoms.

Suppression of Symptoms

Opposing rather than seeking to understand symptoms appears to have three major consequences. First, the manifestation is merely suppressed and reappears in another form. When antibiotic medicine was first introduced more than fifty years ago to treat life-threatening situations, it was dramatically effective. Now, antibiotics are routinely used for conditions where simple immunity may be being compromised – situations which can be due as much to stress and strain as infectivity. This has led to a decrease in the effectiveness of antibiotics and a rise in more serious immunological disorders. Furthermore, there are clear signs that microbial life is resisting and undergoing mutation in response to antibiosis – some hospital operating theatres have had to be closed because antibiotic hygienic measures have been overcome by new strains of microbes.

Avoid the use of antibiotics unless absolutely necessary; 'infectious' conditions indicate that the body is not having sufficient rest.

Recurrence of Symptoms

The second consequence of using allopathic medicines is that symptoms abate, then emerge more severely when treatment is stopped, giving rise to chemical addiction (the body's own chemical production is depressed). The body orders its response to disturbance according to an imbalance in the blood. Pharmaceuticals which arrive directly into the bloodstream are given priority attention, deflecting the blood supply from sites of inflammation. But it is precisely the inflammatory response which allows for the repair of tissues. Thicker, healing blood arrives, the area is intensely irrigated by the lymphatic system and excessive movement is restricted. This creates discomfort but on balance is a small price to pay for usually near perfect repair.

Because anti-inflammatory medicines merely frustrate the body's response to produce less discomfort and do not aid healing, when they are discontinued the body's response is re-established with increased vigour. Perhaps understandably, the offer of more medicine is gladly taken. Unfortunately, within a short time a shift in the body's response is induced: the secretion of natural inflammatory ingredients, known as corticosteroids, decreases. Since the corticosteroids are responsible for the simple wear and tear repairs as well as major requirements, a craving (although it is politely called 'reliance') for anti-inflammatory medicine arises.

The painful congestive condition created by the body's inflammatory response is made bearable by eating little and using hydrotherapy distant from the area of inflammation.

Escalation of Symptoms

A third effect of allopathic medicines, which is associated with the previous one, is that over the long term there are indications that medicine used to manage symptoms eventually contributes towards their continuance. This has been especially confirmed by individuals who have been given medicines to cope with emotional problems.

Pharmaceutical treatment for emotional problems is based on the belief that emotional symptoms are caused by a disorder of the brain's chemistry. This is a rather sophisticated version of the derogatory lay expression for psychological imbalance, 'it's all in your head'. Bizarrely, this treatment is often used in conjunction with an altogether more uncivilized conventional treatment involving giving the brain an electric shock – electro-convulsive therapy (ECT). It would be hard to devise a more punitive, less understanding method of responding to emotional distress.

Naturopathy regards the brain-focused orthodox treatment of emotional symptoms with antidepressive medicines, for example, as a particularly dehumanizing aspect of allopathy. As a treatment, it does not provide a basic requirement of therapy, in that it is incapable of producing any insight for the patient it treats. On the contrary, it tends to magnify emotional problems.

Given the opportunity to express ourselves when we are extremely upset, we tend not to describe the malfunctioning of our brain as our primary distress. Often we observe that only after periods of conventional treatment will someone begin to speak in terms which are neurological, for example, unsteadiness or confusion. Importantly, it is common that while giving the external impression of a less emotional state during conventional therapy, a person will report that their problems simply become internalized, and that the intensity of their feeling increases.

Viewing human nature as basically a blend of robustness and sensitivity, naturopathy observes that using medicines to suppress symptoms, which are essential sensitive effects, is almost guaranteed to increase the energy of the causes behind them. The conventional approach conveniently side-steps this issue, however, by labelling increased manifestation of symptoms as different diseases.

Using suppressive medicines to treat non-life-threatening conditions is counter-productive. When managed naturopathically, symptoms are self-limiting and while they are often inconvenient, the system emerges regenerated.

PAIN

The nervous system is able to distinguish between many levels of sensation – in touch, temperature, intensity and pain. For the majority of these sensations, our response is to adapt gradually or change our posture in a way that will reduce any stress on the body, through an extension of our awareness. But painful stimulation arouses us in a slightly different way in that it is basically alerting us to danger, and requires us to give urgent attention to its cause.

The experience of pain can be actual – measurable in a torn skeletal muscle, the irritation of the intestines or the lack of oxygen to the heart. It can also be emotionally induced from feelings of separation from or loss of a loved one. A combination of the two types of pain can also occur after the amputation of a limb, which is known as 'phantom' pain, whereby the traumatic image of the lost part remains imprinted on our consciousness.

Different parts of the body register different forms of pain and may be insensitive to others. For example it can be shown that the skin is sensitive to cutting and burning, while the stomach is not, and a reduced blood supply to the muscular stomach does not produce the agonizing sensation which is the only proven cause of pain to the heart muscle. It would appear that the message of pain is specialized and appropriate as well as imperative.

For most people, pain is the major symptom and consequently naturopathy considers its interpretation and understanding to be central to therapy. At the same time, while seeking to understand the causes of pain, naturopathy offers management techniques which minimize the discomfort it causes. Although bearing pain is difficult, losing touch with it can make us vulnerable to greater injury.

Perhaps because many orthodox therapies are in themselves

painful, pain-killing medicines have traditionally been offered as therapy. In certain situations, such as during dentistry or childbirth, for example, it would be difficult to imagine anyone withholding pain relief if the patient requested it. The routine use of painkillers is questioned in naturopathy, however, not because pain *has* to be borne, but because using medication to induce insensitivity to pain is not the same as not having pain. Furthermore, with support, painful sensations can be trusted to guide our appropriate responses. It has also been found that at certain times the desire to escape from pain makes for greater discomfort, suggesting that fear may be the most pain-provoking condition.

There are few periods in our existence which are utterly pain-free. Even a comfortable posture becomes uncomfortable if maintained for too long. Moreover, pain may be a feature of normal biological functioning (such as menstruation). To complicate things further, individuals tolerate pain to different degrees and in different ways. What is called pain may represent a multi-layered experience of life. Fear of one type of pain can be associated with the partial awareness of other types which are not fully realized but are still to emerge into consciousness. Without this link, many profound issues in life might remain inaccessible. Studies have recorded that someone's pain from the loss of continuity in a broken limb, for example, can be correlated with a realization of the loss from a fractured relationship. Relaxation, emotional support, selective nourishment and the use of hydrotherapy minimizes pain and creates confidence.

Reserve the use of pain-killing medicine for emergencies. Fear of existing pain is pain-promoting. Paradoxically, fully experiencing pain can be pain-alleviating, if we can give way to tears; the chemical analysis of tears reveals the presence of the body's natural pain-relieving hormones.

LIFE AND DEATH

So accustomed are we to the culture of 'cure until death' in the biomedical system that it is perhaps surprising to learn that the impact of this method on largely preventable disorders such as cardiovascular disease, is relatively small. Professor McKeown has also shown that the triumph over the infectious conditions which decimated the population in former times was a nutritional rather than a clinical success.

Yet we continue to support a biomedicine which is incredibly expensive for the service it provides and operates a system which does not always ensure that the best care is available, and are prepared to undergo untested surgical procedures and consume medicines with known, dangerous side-effects. Even when voices from within biomedicine appeal for a redesign of our medical thinking, consumers are hesitant to support radical changes. Perhaps this is because we crave the image of an all-powerful, infallible medicine, which may help palliate our fear of dying.

Naturopathy contends that the fear of dying is not the same as the fear of death. The latter is probably life-saving since it provides reflexive actions and avoidance behaviours in hazardous circumstances. On the other hand, the fear of dying is a fantasy phobia, which undermines our inner confidence and encourages us to place our faith in external agencies.

Perhaps only in hospice care do we begin to have our deathly fears treated honestly and appropriately. Yet hospices do not benefit from the funding available to other areas of orthodox medicine and these institutions are relatively few in number. It is also interesting to note that this care takes place in a scenario defined as beyond cure. Rather in the same sense that many emotionally disturbed people have stated that one has to become really 'mad' (beyond treatment) before gaining access to a mental institution, it is ironic that we may have to be approaching death before conventional medicine begins to prioritize on our care. Naturopaths suggests that the favourable shift of emphasis which balances cure with care in general medicine has to begin with individual responsiveness to life and death.

Naturopaths do not view death as something which takes place at the end of life but rather as part of an ongoing process, which we experience daily at the microbiological level of our bodies. In fact, our physical continuance requires the successful dying of sufficient cells to stimulate our regeneration. In this sense, life depends on successful dying and this should not be resisted. Conversely, according to the relationship between our cells, it is possible to say that a successful ultimate death is not likely to be the consequence of a medically reliant existence but rather the complement to successful living. Since disorder amongst our cell life contributes towards the most feared diseases of our times, it is vital in naturopathy to cultivate a positive inner attitude towards the concept of death.

Be glad to die daily; extend your life by celebrating the life in your days rather than the days in your life.

4

How Naturopathic Treatment Works

Health is not a 'product' which can be guaranteed by the art of healing; treatment involves manipulation of a patient that is sensitive to their context and to the forces of nature that are struggling to find a new equilibrium in their body.

Hans-Georg Gadamer, German philosopher

NATUROPATHIC TREATMENT IS SAFE, reliable and pleasant, emphasizing the 'treat' in treatment. It is usually given by practitioners, with the active co-operation of the patient, but it is also possible to self-administer by following basic naturopathic principles. This chapter describes the naturopathic consultation process and explains how treatment works with the body's systems.

Naturopathy is not merely a collection of 'natural' remedies. Unlike allopathy, which seeks to overcome individual symptoms through opposition, naturopathy works by supporting normal functioning. It primarily helps to create a restful atmosphere in the body but it can also be gently stimulating. Its methods are based on our present knowledge of anatomy, physiology and psychology but there is also a provision for the unknown, indefinable elements which contribute to the spirit of healing. Particularly recognized is the interdependence of the parts of our being, and there is no attempt to treat disorder as the 'breakdown' of an individual organ. For naturopaths, the manifestations of symptoms suggest disintegration, which requires a positive response; treatment focuses on reintegration, not excision or further polarization.

While preferring to look at disorders within the context of everyday existence, naturopaths are concerned with personal as much as medical history. This is because most symptoms have taken a considerable time to develop the momentum needed to reach our consciousness. Other symptoms may be connected with traumatic events of the past which have been literally buried by our efforts to reassemble our daily lives.

Equally, naturopathic treatment is directed towards the patient's immediate comfort as well as their longer-term interests. Successful treatment initially relieves pressure, which allows for the re-formation of energy and the creation of new patterns of health. Occasionally, treatment may give rise to a slight temporary increase in discomfort for the sake of a more harmonized future but the methods of naturopathy ensure that this is bearable.

CONSULTATION

Consultation is a process whereby people focus upon one another. The consultant 'sees' the patient, while the patient 'goes to see' the consultant. It is a form of witnessing, where the curiosity of the consultant validates the experience of the patient. This is the theme of naturopathic consultation, where the practitioner assumes a therapeutic role in the original Greek sense – as an attendant who *accompanies* the patient.

The naturopath will aim to establish an empathetic, sharing relationship with the patient. This will involve not only seeking to understand the symptoms but being able to communicate understanding in a way that reduces the patient's apprehensions.

Naturopathic consultation is flexible, sometimes taking the form of a detailed interview, at other times simply helping a patient to tell their story. It might be desirable to record readings of blood pressure or weight for future reference or it may seem more appropriate to explore areas of conflict in the family or working environment. Naturopaths will often directly ask how a patient feels about having the symptoms as part of conducting a thorough examination. It is then possible to review together the presenting symptoms within the emerging framework of the patient's life.

From this joint deliberation, the naturopath will endeavour to establish an increase in care, from both introduced therapy and self-applications. An initial, lengthy, consultation may be followed up by therapy sessions and reports on the effects of home treatments.

If a practitioner is not available, it is still possible to employ naturopathy by working intuitively and extending one's knowledge of the human body. A unique form of questionnaire is described in the Appendix, which can assist in self-help as well as in conjunction with practitioner care.

Below is an example of the kind of case record which may be made during consultation. Appreciating the potentially intrusive nature of case recording, questioning may not follow the formal sequence of the case card and the naturopath will encourage the patient to answer in ways which, while maintaining a clinical focus, retain a conversational style.

A

Name, Address & Tel. no. (coded) ....

Presenting Symptoms...

Date of Birth .... Parents .... Marital Status .... Children/Births ....

Health History ....

Medication/Surgery..

....

B

Where Born .... Height .... Weight .... Blood Pressure ....

Immunizations and Vaccinations ....

Sleep .... Exercise/Recreation .... Employment ....

C

B/fast .... Eggs .... Fluids .... Fats ....

Lunch .... Cheese ...... Tea/Coffee/Citrus fruits .... Carbohydrates ....

Dinner .... Meat .... Salt/Sugar .... Salad/Fruit ....

Supper .... Milk .... Tobacco/Alcohol .... Supplement ....

D

Lungs .... Bowels .... Bladder .... Skin .... Menstruation ....

Aches/Pains .... Accidents ....

Joints ankle/knee/hip/wrist/elbow/shoulder..

.... Car/Shoes/Bed   Leg length   Pass moves forward/backwards/left tilt/ right tilt/tortion [turning right then left]

Impressions (coded) ....

The information obtained from section A gives the practitioner an immediate impression of the state of the patient's health. Although a complicated history of disorders can seem clinically impressive, it is often the background features such as age, health of parents and sibling relationships which give an indication of the relative severity of the symptoms being presented.

Naturopaths are concerned about medical history from as far back as the patient can recall. Importance is especially placed on aspects of illness or emotional events which were untreated or trivialized from the patient's point of view.

Section B records measurements which the patient may feel substantiate their symptoms. Recordings are often relative, however, and should not form the basis of a comparison with an ideal; blood-pressure readings, for example, are known to vary depending on who performs the procedure. Practitioners might find it useful to have readings as a baseline for measuring the benefits of some aspects of treatment.

Since nutrition forms the core of naturopathy, section C takes account of detailed aspects of food and eating. Consumption of individual foods (especially the more concentrated, acid-producing types such as proteins), daily amounts of fresh foods, the amount of fluids drunk (in all forms), and use of food supplementation is recorded. The extent to which the common anti-nutrient ingredients, such as salt, appear in the diet, are noted.

It is necessary to discover not only the foods consumed but also how meals are conceived, with whom, at what times and how regularly. There is a tremendous variance in eating practices. Some people eat three formal meals per day, others hardly at all and some, as one practitioner has described, 'eat only one meal per day but take all day to eat it'!

Having become omnivorous, human beings are capable swallowing almost any foodstuff. This is not the same as being able to digest and assimilate its nutrients, of course, and the same holds true for obviously inappropriate foods. Yet naturopaths are not inclined to take literally comments such as 'this food does not agree with me'. A French performing artist has managed over several years to consume, apart from other smaller objects, fifteen supermarket trolleys, six chandeliers but only one light aircraft.

Section D enables the practitioner to rephrase questions about well-being by linking the patient's awareness to any functional problems associated with elimination or mobility. Also, a simple enquiry such as 'Do you have any aches and pains over and above your symptoms?' often illicits helpful information not rated as a priority by the patient.

Finally, when the patient has begun to relax into the consultation, the practitioner will make postural assessments by asking the patient to make gentle spinal stretches and to show how freely they can move their limbs.

Although symptoms may be associated with pathology and the patient's case is essentially a record of disorder, the naturopath aims to make the experience of consultation a conversation about well-being. During this first meeting some supportive therapy will be given, usually in the form of massage and mobilization, and suggestions will be made which will continue the benefits of treatment at home. A follow-up appointment within a short time will be offered, depending on severity of symptoms, allowing the practitioner the opportunity to reflect on the case and the patient to begin some home care.

HOW NATUROPATHY WORKS WITH THE BODY

A written account of the human body inadequately describes how marvellous it is. The traditional method of description, system by system, tends to create a mechanistic impression of a body of many parts. In fact, the body is the result of the development of a threefold layering from a ball of primitive cells, which gives rise to three highly organized systems: skeleton, musculature and circulation; respiration and digestion; and the skin and nerves.

For convenience, organs may also be viewed in groups which have apparently common functions, such as the lungs, kidneys and colon, which create subsystems such as excretion, or the hormonal and circulatory organs which comprise the immune system. The primary structures remain intimately connected throughout life, however, and from a naturopathic point of view, it is neither possible nor desirable to treat one organ in isolation from another. Naturopaths disagree with conventional medical specialization which compartmentalizes disorders. Skin disorders are just as likely to be connected with diet or nervousness as with contact irritants.

The main feature of an organ is that it is not merely a special concentration of cells but that it is 'intelligently organized' by the autonomic nervous system of the brain. The autonomic nerves are ancient, subconscious evolutionary structures and are pre-programmed from millions of years of successful evolution. They ensure an adaptive and energetic life and constantly seek to create circumstances which are most favourable for the individual, whether in the complex extraction of nourishment from food or in controlling the amount of light which enters the eyes.

It is not unreasonable to consider that symptoms are intelligent indications, via the organs, that all is not well autonomically. This invites the sensitive response which characterizes naturopathic treatment, using as a guide the extent to which the patient seems to under- or overuse their body.

NOTE: The professional treatments which follow are for information only, and are not intended to be used for isolated symptomatic experimentation. Home treatments are entirely safe, but where possible use them in conjunction with professional treatment. If naturopathic consultation is unavailable, proceed cautiously with home treatment to build up your confidence. For information on massage treatments used in naturopathy, see *The Complete Illustrated Guide to Massage*, details of which are given in the Recommended Reading section.

THE DIGESTIVE, RESPIRATORY AND ENDOCRINE SYSTEMS

Treatment recognizes the interdependence of digestion and respiration in determining the quality of our blood and hormones.

Life on earth depends on four ingredients – water, air, oxygen-producing plants and the sun's heat. Early naturopathic practitioners were sometimes known as 'sunshine doctors' because they attempted to connect patients with the elemental aspects of their lives. In particular, they emphasized an original definition of nutrition: a process whereby sunlight is transformed into the human body.

When plants grow by harnessing the sun's rays and 'breathing in' carbon dioxide, they contribute oxygen and edible plant material to the environment. Conveniently, animals thrive on oxygen and plant food and, usefully, breathe out carbon dioxide.

Strictly speaking, all creatures are to some degree vegetarian, needing the same fundamental vegetable-sourced nutrients. Although some prefer to take their food material courtesy of another animal's body, it is unusual for a carnivorous animal to eat another carnivore. Although a 'wholefood' approach is generally adopted among meat-eating animals, it is the vitamin- and mineral-rich organ meat which usually constitutes the main part of the meal. Naturopaths point to the inconsistency of the human preference for muscle meat and recommend instead a diet which directly accesses leafy, sun-filled foods.

Nourishment from food is not directly accessible to the body, however. Rather in the same way that a glowing fire is the result of a balance of raw materials and air, so too the body relies on food combined with oxygen for its energy. Adequate respiration is equally as important as food selection. Without oxidization, food is not only underutilized but can become an encumbrance to the body. Taking the fire analogy further, when the fire is not glowing there is the temptation to add more fuel; in the body, when energy is not available, we tend to add more food. In both instances, there comes a time when a clear-out becomes inevitable, which is commonly regarded as 'going off our food'.

Just as the soil is credited with producing the plant, naturopathy contends that it is nutrition, now in the form of blood, which produces the body. Indeed, in contrast to the myriad disease labels which characterize conventional medicine, naturopathy labels only one disease – poor blood. It is the quality of the blood which is responsible for the growth, repair and development of every cell in the body.

Blood is assisted in this majestic rôle by the creation of an endocrine system – an agency of powerful glandular secretions, known as *hormones*, strategically sited throughout the body. Hormones are unique in our make-up, in that they act not only on behalf of the individual body but for humanity as a whole. The word 'hormone' means 'I urge' and we often find their prompting irresistible, despite our personal convictions. It is the foetus's hormone which stimulates the mother to begin birthing; it is the resonance between the complementary sex hormones which creates new human life; it could be said that it is the withdrawal of the repair hormone which ends our life. Of all the

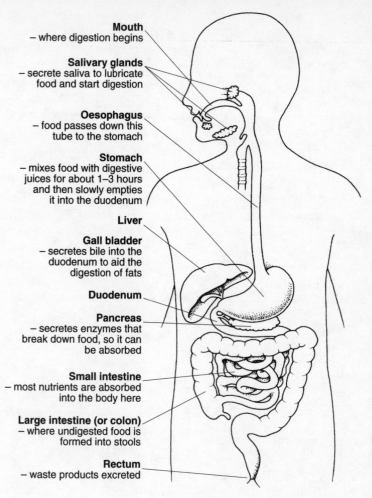

Mouth
– where digestion begins

Salivary glands
– secrete saliva to lubricate food and start digestion

Oesophagus
– food passes down this tube to the stomach

Stomach
– mixes food with digestive juices for about 1–3 hours and then slowly empties it into the duodenum

Liver

Gall bladder
– secretes bile into the duodenum to aid the digestion of fats

Duodenum

Pancreas
– secretes enzymes that break down food, so it can be absorbed

Small intestine
– most nutrients are absorbed into the body here

Large intestine (or colon)
– where undigested food is formed into stools

Rectum
– waste products excreted

Figure 3   The digestive system

organizations within us, the endocrine is the most subtle and in both Eastern and conventional Western Medicine, it has been regarded as the 'spiritual' system of the body.

Professional Treatment

Diet is assessed to take into account the patient's age, occupation and recreations and their family's eating history. The patient receives guidance in breathing to encourage them to breathe out effortlessly for twice as long as it takes to breathe in, then to

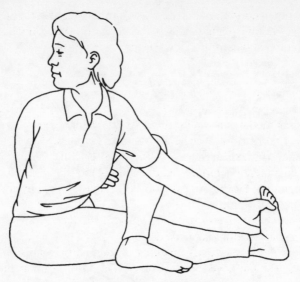

Figure 4   Practise hatha yoga

graduate to holding the breath for a few seconds between inhaling and exhaling. It is important that this is learned with a practitioner, since adjusting one's breathing pattern can be initially disorienting.

Massage is also given, which focuses on the spinal areas adjacent to the endocrine glands.

Home Treatment

Eat green leafy vegetables daily. Practise hatha yoga, a system which co-ordinates respiratory movements with postures designed to massage the hormonal glands. Be alert to the use of medicines which mimic the body's own hormones. Since your own hormones function as an orchestra, long-term use of substitutes may seriously disrupt their natural harmony.

CASE STUDY: *DIGESTIVE DISORDER – indigestion and overweight*

Bill, aged 50, married, a retailer

Bill's diet was becoming very limited since there were few foods which he could eat without experiencing discomfort. At the same time, he found that he was gaining weight. Having tried various dieting regimes without success, he heard about food-combining and consulted a naturopath for advice.

Examination

Although not clinically obese, Bill's weight suggested that his intake of food was in excess of his needs. His indigestion took the form of pain in his stomach soon after eating and in his lower abdomen within an hour. An analysis of Bill's normal meals showed a preponderance of cooked milky foods, bread, fish, meat and potatoes. He did not eat many vegetables since they appeared to increase the pain.

When his indigestion started early in the day, he survived by eating snacks throughout the day.

He was always the first member of the family to finish a meal. He was self-employed and found that running a small business was very time-consuming. Consequently, he was usually the first to leave the table and would immediately continue with work he had brought home.

His general health was otherwise good but he was aware that he was not getting much outdoor exercise.

Treatment

Indigestion is the most prevalent male eating disorder. It is thought to be the most under-reported symptom, since many men are under the impression that indigestion is normal. Typically, only when the condition produces acute pain is professional help sought. Even then it is commonly from a pharmacist rather than a doctor, since remedies for indigestion account for the majority of over-the-counter medicines available.

Evidence shows that even moderate excess weight, if un-checked, leads to obesity. Being technically overweight imposes strain at many levels of health, including joint strain, high blood pressure and respiratory problems. The risk of accident at home and work has also been shown to increase. Ultimately, obesity reduces life expectancy considerably.

It was explained to Bill that the digestive system was, in evolutionary terms at least, a most robust part of the body. Therefore, symptoms of indigestion were likely to represent the unsuitability of foods or eating habits. His immediate pain may have been from an inappropriate food combination, while later discomfort might have reflected incomplete digestion from the earlier stages.

Both excess weight and indigestion can be complications arising from unacknowledged distress. Foods eaten when emotionally upset are not well utilized by the body. Often starchy, comforting foods are chosen or eaten in the form of 'nibbles', as a displacement activity rather than to fuel activity. Also, the chemical activity of digestion is depressed, as are its smooth muscular movements, during times of stress.

Emotional states associated with digestive disorders are characterized in everyday expressions: such as 'I am sick of . . .', 'I can't stomach . . .' and 'belly-aching'.

Bill first task was to replace starchy foods with raw vegetables, such as chopped carrots or celery for nibbling. It was explained that raw vegetables were more digestible than cooked and that the main point was to dissipate nervous tension rather than get energy. The following was suggested:

- He should have a simple fruit breakfast, as much as he wanted, and a hot drink.
- Main meals should begin with small raw salad, and there should be no drinking with meals.
- He should avoid rich food combinations – starches with fats, such as buttered dishes, and fried foods – and limit eggs to three per week.
- He should eat no salt or spices other than a little black pepper.
- There was no limit to the size of his portions, but he should stop eating when he was satisfied.
- He should try to become the last to finish eating.

Comment

This approach worked well for Bill. He immediately felt more comfortable during a meal, and his lower abdominal pain gradually disappeared. Although he was not consciously reducing foods, he lost weight quickly, then more over a longer term. Sometimes if he is was busy, he skipped a meal and nibbled raw vegetables while he worked. He felt less strained by his business and he looked forward to a relaxing meal.

THE SKELETAL SYSTEM

Naturopathic treatment promotes posture, which is balance between the bones.

Although the word 'skeleton' literally means 'dried up', in the living body our bones glisten. The framework which is our skeleton is made up of cells, which in the interior of bones are relatively soft, becoming rigid only towards the outside. The surface of the bone is finished in a polished, delicate membrane to allow the inter-passage of nerves and blood vessels.

The term 'lazy-bones' is one of the greatest physical misnomers. Bones are extraordinarily busy. They are light yet strong, achieving an amazing load-bearing capacity through their hollowish structure, rather as a rolled-up piece of paper can support an object many times its weight. Bones look after themselves extremely well. It is remarkable, for example, that they are able to grow without disturbing the body. This is achieved by specialist bone cells which excavate the inner bone while others lay down new cells on the exterior. Using a similar method, if it is deranged by fracture, a bone will rearrange a poor external alignment by gnawing away at the jagged edge and infilling to establish a smoother finish.

The skeleton is not merely a scaffolding for the body, it is also an immensely versatile construction. It is fabulously jointed to allow for the sophisticated movements which put our physical potential beyond that found anywhere else in nature. The joints of our limbs are extremely flexible but the fused parts of the adult skeleton, the skull and pelvis, were plastic in comparison at the time of our birth. The spine is the pivot around which the whole body articulates. It is made up of thirty-three separate bones but because each is multi-faceted, the spine of even the most unfit person makes over a hundred jointed movements. Joints allow the ends of bones to glide past each other but when pressure increases around a joint, the bones may become inflamed.

Treatment

Naturopathic treatment concentrates on the relationships between bones, especially two vulnerable areas of the spine – the neck and skull, and the joints of the base of the spine with

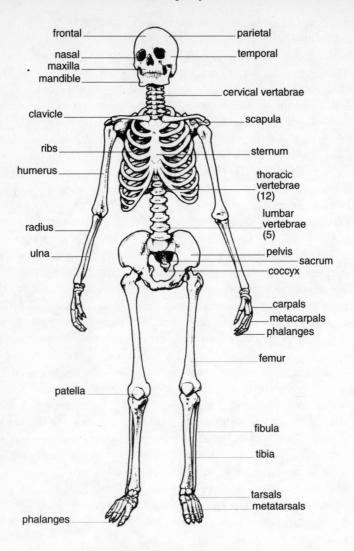

Figure 5   The human skeleton

the pelvis. Apart from being points of strain in our upright posture, the spinal nerves which issue from these joints influence important organic functions in the body and are sensitive to joint inflammation. Attention will also be given to relieving pressure on the spine from the unremitting, compressing effects of gravity.

Professional Treatment for the Neck Region

In the neck region, increased pressure may be reflected in distress to the head, heart, lungs and digestion and loss of strength in the arms. After neck massage with the patient lying face upwards, the head will be slowly rolled, tilted sideways and rotated to each side. Whichever side offers most resistance will be retreated. Finally, holding the base of the skull and beneath the jaw, while the patient exhales the practitioner will gently apply traction to release pressure from the weight of the head on the neck.

Home Treatment for the Neck Region

Self-massage is given by placing a towel behind the neck and creating gentle friction by pulling the ends of the towel from left to right. After lying down with a pillow under the knees, the towel is then rolled up and placed under the neck, close to the shoulders. This will help keep movements smooth and cushion the neck against overstretching. The same slow rolling, tilting and rotating movements are done, twice to the tighter

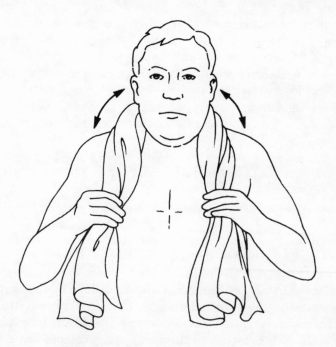

Figure 6   Self-massage for the neck region

side. Self-stretching of the neck is achieved by relaxing the jaw and breathing deeply.

Professional Treatment for the Lower Spine

Low back pressure is exacerbated by our sitting posture, which abuses the pelvis, and the tendency to favour one-sidedness, which twists the lower back. Problems manifested from this include pelvic inflammation, lower abdominal pain, radiating pain in the legs and varicosity.

The patient lies on their back and one knee is flexed up towards the chest and drawn across to the opposite side of the body. The legs are then extended over a pillow and the shoulder on the opposite side is rotated while the pelvis remains fixed. The stiffer sides are re-treated.

For traction, the practitioner raises both legs by the feet and while the patient holds the couch above the head, swings the legs from side to side, then slowly pulls straight down in line with the spine.

Home Treatment for the Lower Spine

The first-aid recovery position, lying face down with one leg brought up alongside the chest (*see* Figure 14, p. 87), can be adopted, keeping the leg well up. Squatting from a standing position is also an option, with the feet flat if possible, turning the shoulders away from the stiffer side. Hanging by the arms, keeping the feet on the floor, while rotating the hips to each side unwinds the low back and exerts a controlled traction.

THE MUSCULAR SYSTEM

Treatment helps maintain positive tension – 'tone' – in the muscles.

The appearance of rippling beneath the skin gave rise to the word muscle, which is derived from the Latin *musculos*, 'little mouse'. Some muscles are like rather big mice, like those of the legs, but there are also minuscule ones such as the erectors which are attached to every hair of the body.

The muscular system is faithful to the commands of the motor nerves, which relay action signals issuing from the brain. The muscles can also send messages back to the brain through sensory nerves which detect pressure, which contributes towards our understanding of our environment. Some of this activity is conscious, in the sense that we appear to be in control of it, and indeed this is true for the muscles which move our skeleton. We do not directly control the muscles of the inner workings of the body, however, for rather obvious reasons.

In fact, the unconscious controls are able to override the conscious, so that we are often aware of excessive tension in our skeletal muscles without having 'ordered' it. An everyday example of this is when an emergency requires us to lift a heavy object or run very fast; we find ourselves successful out of all proportion to our normal strength. This indicates that the origin of raised skeletal muscular tension is perception of danger. Naturopaths are careful to record the tension of the consciously controlled muscles. Not only is this a guide to general fitness but if it is found to be inconsistent with normal use of the body, it is a clear indication of the state of tension in the organs.

Extreme tension is an everyday requirement of the body, from rising up from bed in the morning to expelling a sneeze, from raising our blood pressure to digesting our main meal. When we are healthy there is a rhythmic exchange, where high tension alternates with low, and one part of the body relaxes while another gears up. If hypertension is maintained beyond our immediate requirements, through fear or apprehension, however, this can create far-reaching disturbances in the body.

Treatment

Rhythmic massage is given to the muscular system since muscles themselves are the body's own massage machinery. Treatment concentrates on relieving the cycle which occurs when a perceived threat leads to increased tension, leading in turn to a feedback from the muscles which orders up more tension. Muscles are also responsive to the mechanical influence of massage which helps recondition their structure from repetitive use and habitual posture.

Professional Treatment for the Back
Rigidity in the back muscles restricts the movement of the entire body and eventually produces severe discomfort. Massage is

given lying face down or leaning forward over a pillow. The large muscles which connect the spine with the head, shoulders and pelvis are treated first, then the muscles which lie the entire length of the back from head to tail are lengthened by squeezing and stretching. When the back muscles are in spasm, the abdominal muscles will also be massaged.

Home Treatment for the Back

You should not attempt to massage the back muscles with your own hands, except perhaps for simple frictions which can be achieved by pulling a towel across the back of the neck, across the shoulders or behind the waist. Deeper effects are gained by short (five minute) hot baths and the slow rotational movements of yoga.

Professional Treatment for the Arms and Legs

Modern life discourages the full movement of the arm and leg muscles, particularly activity which utilizes the ball and socket arrangement of the shoulder and hip joint. Alternate compression and release strokes are given from the extremity towards the trunk. The muscles are 'rung out' and deep draining movements are made towards each joint. The joints are fully flexed and extended. Vigorous upper arm massage is known to decrease tension in the heart and lungs by reflexing unconscious controls.

Home Treatment for the Arms and Legs

Lying on your back, with head and shoulders slightly raised on pillows, hold one leg up while squeezing the muscles towards the trunk. The inverted position, combined with draining strokes, reduces pressure and tiredness in the muscles.

Professional Treatment for Invigoration

Massage can be overstimulating if prolonged, but brief, intense treatment is useful after being confined to bed or if you continually have to travel on long journeys. The massage is brisk, especially over the spine. Percussion strokes, which involve repetitive tapping, or lightly chopping, are applied to the limbs and the muscles are rhythmically stretched and released.

Home Treatment for Invigoration

Contrast hydrotherapy, which is massage using hot and cool water, is the easiest and most effective invigorating self-massage. Using a spray, give your body thirty seconds of hot water then thirty of cool, six times, always ending with cool. Wrap yourself in towels and rest.

Professional Treatment for Relaxation

The influence of massage has sometimes been misunderstood because of an imagined relaxed and helpless effect. In fact, the opposite is true. Excessive effort is wasteful and certainly inefficient and is likely to be the greatest contributor to weakness, whereas massage not only helps liberate but positively transform hypertension.

Vigorous massage is given at first to the back, followed by slow, deep strokes directed to the limbs and neck. Oil may be used to deflect the pressure of the strokes. The muscles are slowly stretched to comfortable limits. Breathing movements, especially emphasizing exhalation, may be given to increase oxygen to loosening muscles. Aromatic essences known to affect mood may be added to the massage oil.

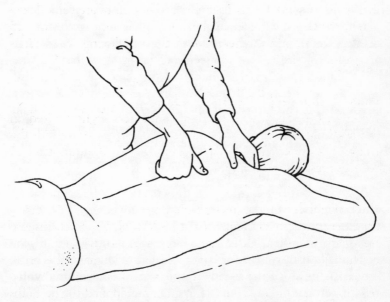

Figure 7   Professional treatment for relaxation

Home Treatment for Relaxation

Lying down on a padded surface, fold your arms and cross your ankles. Slowly rock your hips and shoulders from side to side, at first in unison, then in opposition. Then make a cushion with your hands behind your head, while drawing your feet close to your hips. Leaning forward and drawing your left knee to your chest, aim your right elbow towards your knee. Repeat this using the opposite limbs, then both arms and legs at the same time. Movements may be complemented with a hydrotherapy which involves placing a cool cloth around the waist, wrapped in warm towelling, for a surprisingly soothing relaxant.

THE CIRCULATORY SYSTEM

Treatment relieves congestion and encourages return flow through the veins and lymphatic vessels.

The circulatory system is responsible for distributing nutritious blood to the body and collecting waste from our cells. It achieves this through the pumping action of the heart and three sets of tubes, the arteries and veins and the lesser-known lymphatic vessels.

The arterial and venous arrangements are complementary. Major arteries subdivide until they are just one cell wide to deliver blood, and the veins start at first from each cell, increasing in size as they converge to bring blood back to the heart. Since some of the fluidity of our blood is lost in this process and the cells themselves are suspended in a watery environment, the interstitial fluid, it is vital that escaped fluid (lymph) from the blood vessels is recovered. If it is not, and this is sometimes the case in severely degenerated circulatory systems, the body literally fills up with water. A temporary example of this is seen if one has to sleep, during the night particularly, in a sitting position. By morning it is difficult to put shoes on due to water retention in the feet. A simple movement of the leg muscles remedies the situation in a healthy body, and this is the clue to maintaining an efficient lymphatic system.

The lymph travels in tubes very similar to those of the veins but crucially, since the escaped water contains cleansing white cells from the blood and is contaminated by use by the inflammatory processes of the body, it is periodically filtered and

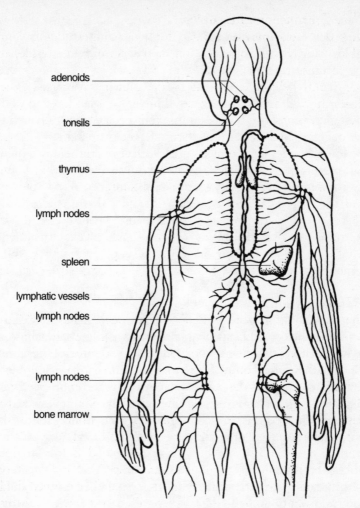

adenoids

tonsils

thymus

lymph nodes

spleen

lymphatic vessels

lymph nodes

lymph nodes

bone marrow

Figure 8   The lymphatic system

the debris combusted in structures called nodes. The back of the
knee, under the arm, beneath the jaw and at the back of the skull
are places where the nodes are easily felt when active. The
'busier' the area of the body, the more obvious is the functioning
of the nodes, increasing in size and temperature around
menstruation or near the site of an injury.

By the time the lymph is recovered into whole blood in the
large veins near the heart, it has been thoroughly cleansed. While
naturopathic treatment has much to offer the circulatory system as

a whole, it is specifically concerned with encouraging effective lymphatic return and supporting the function of the nodes.

Treatment

Rarely in modern life do we sufficiently make use of our musculature and it is estimated that up to 20 per cent of lymph is not reabsorbed daily, because of inadequate stimulation. This is experienced as sluggishness and weariness and explains the debilitating effects of a long journey, from sitting doing nothing.

When a node's activity increases, it is tender, it may pulsate and the muscles nearby become stiffened. All this helps focus energy in the node but it undeniably creates discomfort. Naturopathy strongly rejects conventional medical treatment which suppresses the node for the sake of pain relief, while disabling its vital cleansing role.

Professional Treatment

Helping maintain good muscle tone through massage directly contributes to an efficient lymphatic system. Lymphatic massage of underactive areas consists of gentle, superficial stroking, combined with a smooth continuous pressure stroke ('deep draining') towards the heart, then moving outwards and working back again from the extremities. Like the veins, the lymph vessels also benefit from deep inspirational breathing, which may form part of treatment or be a longer-term benefit of massage.

Home Treatment

The distress associated with inflamed nodes can be minimized by the simplification of the diet and the use of compresses. Eating raw food or consuming only juices tends to decrease the intensity of inflammation when combined with rest. A compress positioned around the node produces a relieving self-massage.

THE NEUROLOGICAL SYSTEM

Treatment directly influences nervous action through the application of pressure massage and gentle manipulation.

The centre of the nervous system is the brain, although it would be more accurate to say human beings possess 'brains', which we have collected over the course of our evolution. The oldest of these is the brain stem, a structure associated with acute perception and instinctive action. This area is sometimes called the 'old brain', as it functions similarly in all animals. The cerebellum, situated at the back of the skull, is also an organ we have in common with other animals, but given its role in the choreography of movement, it is uncommonly large in humans.

The largest part of the brain is the cerebrum, or cerebral cortex, a bundle of nerves which develop around the brain stem. It has such potential for growth that in order for it to be accommodated within the skull, it has to fold over and over into the convolutions which characterize its surface appearance. The cerebrum is specifically human, containing all the knowledge developed from birth. It is not, proportionately, the largest cerebrum of all animals – horses and dolphins have more developed convolutions – nor has it increased in size over thousands of years. What distinguishes our modern brain is the shape of the cortex, which has extended forward, just behind the forehead, into what is termed the frontal lobe. This part is associated with our moral consciousness.

Not only do we have different component brains but the cerebrum and cerebellum are actually composed of two mirrored aspects. The cognition within each side of the cerebrum has been found to be qualitatively different, the left side specializing in logical and the right in abstract thought. Furthermore, the nerves which issue from the right cerebrum and cerebellum cross over lower down in the brain to control the left side of the body and vice versa. Although a great deal has been discovered about the intricacies of the brain's functioning, the rationale for this eccentric arrangement between the hemispheres has not been satisfactorily explained.

The brain's motor nerves predominate in our muscular tissues, while those relaying messages back from the surfaces of the internal organs and the skin are the sensory nerves. Occasionally one nerve possesses both qualities. The spinal column provides a safe conduit for their passage, and they branch symmetrically from the spaces between the vertebrae. A separate set of nerves, the twelve pairs of cranials, leave the brain just beneath the skull and innervate the head and face. One pair deviates to wander down through the trunk, as an agent of parasympathy,

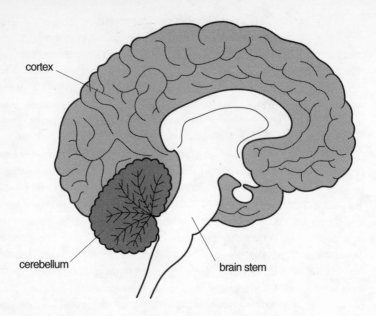

Figure 9   The brain, showing the relative structures of the cortex, brain stem and cerebellum

relaxing conditions of overexcitement. These are the celebrated vagus nerves.

Treatment

Nerves are very responsive to external pressure. Naturopaths apply slow deep pressures to relax nervous tension and give quicker, stimulating contact to encourage activity.

Professional Treatment

Vigorous friction of the skin supplies stimulation to the peripheral nerves, which is often denied in modern life. This creates a reflex action, producing a calming influence on the central nervous system.

Reprogramming of the cerebellum after loss of confidence and poise from an accident or emotional trauma is achieved by passive movement of the body, including joint articulations following massage. The parasympathizing influence of the vagus nerves can be induced by softly massaging adjacent muscles at the side of the neck.

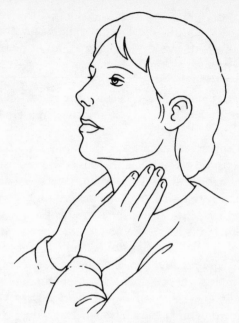

Figure 10   Activating the vagus nerves

Home Treatment

The stimulation of peripheral nerves can be achieved by alternating hot and cool showers or by a friction glove or body brush. Cerebellum activity can be stimulated by patiently learning a new activity, or practising stylized, statuesque movements such as Tai Chi. The vagus nerves can be activated by contact through the neck muscles and via reflex action by touching the face. This is sometimes observed by the way we spontaneously rub the side of the neck when we are under stress. Simple facial massage is equally effective, especially if the palms are pressed lightly against the eyeballs for a few seconds.

THE ELIMINATIVE SYSTEMS

Treatment offsets the suppressive influence of modern life on elimination.

The principal eliminative routes are the skin, the lungs, the kidneys and the large intestine. Through these organs the body loses the by-products of metabolism.

The skin disposes of excess heat via conduction, convection, radiation and perspiration; the lungs exhale water and carbon dioxide; the kidneys release water and acids from the blood; the large intestine recycles water and eliminates undigested matter and worn-out blood cells. Although there is a widespread notion that retained waste material can become toxic, it would be more accurate to say that it has the potential to interfere with the body's functioning rather than contaminate it.

Naturopathy observes that the body eliminates wastes skilfully and relatively effortlessly – unless there is an accumulation from overconsumption or pollution, or when the body has become exhausted. At such times emergency elimination become necessary and the inner skins, which line the body organs, become hyperactive. Since this lining is a mucous membrane, it may run (a cold), become sticky (a cough) or loosen (diarrhoea or heavy menstruation). Naturopathy agrees with the conventional view that where there is no apparent reason for eliminative symptoms externally, their cause is probably invisible. However, while infections are the favoured conventional agency, naturopaths are more likely to suggest 'emotions', and this produces diametrically opposed treatments.

Since eliminative products are destined to leave the body, naturopathy finds it logical to help facilitate rather than suppress their exit. Not only that, but the processes of emergency elimination which medical treatment frustrates, such as increased temperature and immobilization, are observed by naturopaths to be helpful in themselves.

Professional Treatment

Between twenty-four and forty-eight hour's absolute rest will be recommended, and a short juice fast may be advised, especially if the appetite is low.

Superficial but vigorous massage of the skin will not only encourage the circulation but relieve the strain on the internal eliminative surfaces, making for more ease generally.

Hydrotherapies, such as foot bathing to relieve headache, neck compresses for painful nodes or waist compresses to enable sleep, will be applied.

Home Treatment

If raised temperature persists or the chest becomes congested or bowel movements increase, for more than twenty-four hours, reduce your food intake to fruits and vegetables, mostly raw. This will release digestive energy for eliminative work and reduce the intensity of symptoms. Also rest during the day and go to sleep early at night. Use a waist compress or bathe your hands and feet in cool water to become more comfortable for sleep, and decrease, or preferably eliminate, social contact. Avoid newspapers and serious TV. If you feel inclined, read your favourite author.

5

Naturopathic Care for Adults

Practitioner: 'What you need is relaxation, foot massage, relationship counselling, beansprouts, no coffee, no television and no fun – and you really need to pull yourself together!'

New Patient (thinks): 'All I said was I had a bit of a headache'.

ADULTS WHO PRESENT for treatment are generally of two types. There are those suffering acute conditions who have been accustomed to naturopathic care within the family or who are in a chronic state and whose conventional treatment has proved ineffective. There is also another population, of 'walking unwell', who are perhaps seeking a deeper understanding of their symptoms, who may be attracted to naturopathy's benefits but have misgivings about the 'demands' made by treatment. This chapter is written primarily with this latter group in mind. For the sake of clarity, the application of treatment for women, men and for older adults will be discussed separately.

LIFESTYLE

Life expectancy, which is often held to be *the* measure of health, has increased dramatically in the West over the past hundred years. In the UK, for example, it has nearly doubled. With the provision of clean water and improved hygiene, fewer infants die than before but it is the proportion of older people in the population which is growing fastest. World-wide, by the year 2020, the over sixty-five age group is expected to double. This is generally agreed to be a benefit of medical technology, although the quality of extended life has been debated. Apparently, very few people presently die from old age.

Epidemiologists predict that the world faces an explosion in 'lifestyle illnesses', fuelled by pollution, poor diet and longer living. This will take the form of dramatic increases in lingering but potentially fatal disorders of the circulatory, digestive and respiratory systems, as well as incapacitating diseases of the muscles and skeleton. Such conditions are also associated with psychological distress, depression and confusion. Since life expectancy is set to rise, naturopathy stresses the need to approach illness rationally but delicately and compassionately if treatment is to make a significant impression on people's customs and habits.

The 'Child'

Children are not 'little adults' but it has not escaped the attention of clinicians that within each adult there exists a 'child'. Patients often speak of an inner vulnerable presence, sometimes of a tender age, which in spite of life's outer achievements, still retains the insecurities of earlier times. Although it is acknowledged, respecting this immaturity is not a feature of the conventional approach to ill-health. Indeed, the misinterpretation of the 'child's' expression can lead to a psychiatric diagnosis and a severely restraining treatment. In contrast, naturopaths find that treatment is much more effective if the patient's 'child' is allowed expression in consultation.

Ironically, classical terminology, high-tec diagnostic equipment and the theory of 'infection' appeal directly to the 'child' – indeed, some have suggested this as the real reason for the popularity of biomedicine. But the 'child' finds conventional treatment methods superficial and unsatisfying. Driven from the original part of the brain, symptoms require a deeper response than prescriptive medicines and patch-up surgery.

The effects of illness may provide the opportunity for legitimate regression in the adult world. When one is aching, fevered or weakened, even the busiest, most important schedules may have to be interrupted, perhaps cancelled. Decisions are postponed, and even trying to think becomes impossible. The very act of expressing discomfort when one is ill can give voice to the strain and pain of the responsibilities imposed on the inner world which the 'child' shares. However well intentioned, the way in which medical treatment is typically given tends to cut short the valuable time spent in stress-relieving regression. The extended time available to be with one's 'child' if one is chronically ill in older age, on the other hand, may not be so useful.

Treatment

The simplistic notion of being 'struck down' with illness is at odds with the rational approach of naturopathy. While the definition of chronic illness is the mismanagement of acute conditions, the extent to which acute illnesses are experienced is seen as a reflection of childhood. If the eliminative system of the child has been supported rather than suppressed, most adult illnesses will be of short duration, and abrupt in beginning and end. Occasionally symptoms may be intense but the patient will feel the benefit of being ill and be emotionally refreshed.

The illness pattern of an adult should be predictable unless they are heavily medicated. As we have seen, the overuse of medical treatment gives rise to a condition known as iatrogenesis. First used by orthodox commentators, this term has also been used to explain the crowded doctor's waiting room and the shortage of hospital beds. It is estimated that up to 25 per cent of repeat consultations and readmissions are due to prescribing errors. Naturopathic treatment begins by instigating a 'wash-out' period through an eliminative diet in such cases, and it may take some time before the full benefits of treatment are experienced.

Naturopathy is realistic in admitting that certain human conditions appear to be beyond the scope of treatment. After many years of conventional work researching individual diseases, however, clinicians are nearer to an understanding that the object of research should encompass not only the disease process but also the patients themselves. The naturopathic consultation provides this in the form of single case research and the discussion which follows draws on general conclusions from a wide range of practice. Examples of commonly presented problems are given. Treatments are safe to try, but it is always preferable to have professional guidance. Practice experience indicates that most benefit will be gained from a treatment which meets with initial resistance.

Asthma

Breathing is commonly disturbed by inflammation of the respiratory passages, which gives rise to well-known disorders, depending on which part is involved – rhinitis, laryngitis and bronchitis. Asthma occurs when the subdivisions of the bronchial tree, the arterioles, become obstructed and it becomes difficult to exhale.

The increasing incidence of asthma has been viewed as an allergic response to airborne substances and pollutants. Urban air contains a cocktail of industrial and transport emissions. In the countryside, crop spraying and even the natural pollens from plants are thought to provoke allergy. Conditions in modern, sealed, air-conditioned homes are also believed to favour respiratory reactions.

Dietary theories to explain asthma revolve around sensitivity to concentrated foods, which can cause excessive mucus production. Cow's milk is often found to be a trigger in allergy testing, and asthma is thought to be a result of its premature introduction to children's diet. Other ingredients which have been discovered to aggravate an established asthmatic condition include table salt, food preservatives and alcohol.

Naturopathy finds an exclusively allergic rationale for asthma too narrow and passive for such dynamic symptoms, which often amount to fighting for breath.

Although a serious breathing condition, asthma rarely is a fatal condition. Nor is it always disabling. Indeed, many top-class athletes have been successful despite being asthmatic. Naturopathy prefers to consider asthma not as a disorder, but as a way of breathing. In this sense, it can still be described as an allergic response, but expressing a more profound intolerance.

Asthma can manifest in children, including the very young. Although there is an assumption that the condition may be 'outgrown', in adulthood it is often seen in the outwardly mature, accomplished individual. Observation suggests that overcoming asthma requires emotional as well as physical development.

During an asthmatic episode, the bronchioles within the lungs are in spasm. Although it is complicated by the presence of thick mucus, naturopaths understand this to come from an underlying tension. Because of the childhood associations of asthma, this tension is thought to belong to feelings of insecurity.

75

The example of the successful athletes suggests that the reassurances sought by an asthmatic are not of the external world. Rather, it hints at the inner person, who finds it difficult to compete emotionally.

As so often with symptoms, the acute episode merely serves to illustrate the underlying condition. During bronchial spasm, not only is the individual unable to speak, they can hardly breathe out at all. Yet the purpose of the symptoms is fulfilled. In such an obvious state of distress, a person becomes the centre of attention. Naturopathy's view of asthma as fundamentally an emotional condition recommends self-treatment, as well as the practitioner's help in showing how to cope with acute situations.

Treatment
- Experiment with ways of 'ventilating' problems and tensions – self-expression without necessarily seeking to solve.
- Lie down and check whether your chest or abdomen rises on

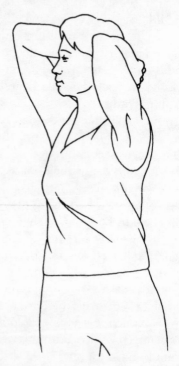

Figure 11   Exercise with movements that involve arm-raising

inhalation. If only the abdomen does, learn to raise the chest too, and vice versa. Practice breathing out for a longer time than it takes to breathe in.

- Exercise with movements that involve arm-raising.
- Use your voice creatively: sing or read poetry out loud.
- Preferably do the above in the company of others.
- A yoga class is an ideal way of achieving this. Yoga is also taught under personal supervision, with due regard for individual requirements.
- Follow nutritional guidelines which will lessen catarrhal tendencies – reducing dairy products, salt and wheat – and possibly minimize the severity of an acute episode.
- Splash your face with cold water throughout the day.
- Bathe your upper arms in hot water if you sense the onset of an acute episode. If it endures use alternate hot and cold compresses on the back of the neck.

NATUROPATHY FOR WOMEN

Period Pain

From menarche to menopause the lining of the uterus is built up, maintained and discarded in a continuous process, which is evidenced in its eliminative phase by the period. In assessing period disorders it is necessary to remember that this lining contains a mucous membrane, a surface the body uses for general elimination.

Many theories having been advanced for period pain, including hormonal derangement. The suggested conventional advice for period pain is radical – the contraceptive pill, childbirth or surgical removal of the womb. Naturopathy concurs with the latest findings in conventional research, which explain that in the preparation for the period the associated vascular system becomes engorged, causing cramp locally and nervous irritation which is referred pain to the spine. Three factors exacerbate this to give greater discomfort: lack of fitness (tone) in the pelvic muscles; low back tension (lordosis), which tips the pelvis forward and impedes blood flow; and systemic catarrh (mucous) from dietary and respiratory disorders.

The period also allows for a loosening 'birthing rehearsal' of the pelvic ligaments, so a certain amount of discomfort is explainable at the front (pubis) and back (sacrum) of the pelvis. General activities, such as bending over may increase the strain (a reason for not washing your hair from a standing position).

Treatment

- Daily, not just during the period, squat with your knees flexed and apart in a bath of 6 inches of cool water. Splash alternately between the legs and to the lower abdomen ten times; the water will not feel cold after the first few splashes. Place a towel around your shoulders to keep warm; do not inhibit any vocalizing – it encourages deep breathing.
- From mid-cycle until after the period, practise inverting your hips as in a yoga shoulder-stand for one minute or lie on an inclined bed. Make toe, ankle and knee movements. It is perfectly safe to invert the pelvis during your period, but be careful to avoid neck or back strain when recovering.
- Reduce your consumption of all liquids by 50 per cent. Avoid salt and decrease your consumption of milk products. Do activities which raise breathing movements to the upper chest.
- For relief during a period, sit in cold water for extended times – up to five minutes. Rest afterwards with a comfortably hot water bottle against your lower back (not your abdomen).

Birthing

Although it is never technically classified as such, in recent times giving birth has been treated as a medical emergency. Just as the practice of breastfeeding was lost for a generation or two through hospitalization, directed births meant that mothers were considered to be unprepared for delivery unless they were shaved, irrigated, gassed and sometimes tied down. At one point it was thought that routinely introducing artificial hormones into the mother's bloodstream might regulate labour.

Fewer births take place in hospital now, although it is sometimes hard to arrange home delivery for a first birth. Midwives are increasingly the managers of hospital births and aim to create a relaxed atmosphere with technical intervention only as safety requires.

CASE STUDY: 4th PREGNANCY COMPLICATION – *'essential hypertension'*

Jayne, aged 35, married and a parent

Jayne was three months pregnant with her fourth child. Births one and two had minor complications but the main feature of the pregnancies was high blood pressure. Obstetricians diagnosed an 'essential hypertension' and advised her against having further children. Despite this, with the aid of some home research on preparation for birth, a successful third pregnancy ensued. However, during her fourth pregnancy, which she welcomed, Jayne became exhausted and sought naturopathic consultation.

Examination
Jayne was positive but tense and tired, and had varicosity of the legs which were slightly painful. Her blood pressure was normal. Otherwise the pregnancy was proceeding well. Jayne's concern was that if her blood pressure rose to an unacceptable level she would be required to spend time in bed during her pregnancy.

Treatment
Initially, the shoulders and neck were massaged to help reduce tension. Cool water splashes on the legs were recommended to relieve pressure on the varicose veins.

Jayne was encouraged to continue her favoured exercise, walking, and she was reminded to raise her feet and do toe exercises while sitting, even if she was not fully resting.

She was able to attend treatment regularly, up to and beyond the trouble-free birth of her fourth child. She used the sessions to focus on relaxation and 'switch off' mentally from family and medical concerns. Having found the time for herself, she was able to keep in a more relaxed state than during previous pregnancies.

Comment
Jayne's case illustrates how easily, even for an experienced mother, pregnancy can become a medical issue. In this instance, obstetricians were rightly concerned that an escalating blood pressure might result in pre-eclampsia, a condition which can threaten the baby. For Jayne, however, enforced bed rest would almost certainly have guaranteed an increase in blood pressure.

With no established hypertensive medicines acceptable during pregnancy, complete rest is the conventional treatment. Although in general treatment rest is highly favoured in naturopathy, for an active pregnant mother a more mobile approach can be recommended.

The Birth Pool

A novel introduction which naturopathy supports is a warm-water birth pool. This provides a hydrotherapy environment which has many advantages during labour. If hospitals do not possess a pool, staff are usually amenable to a rented one being brought in, if they are advised in advance. The advantages of a birth pool are:

- If it is used at home during pregnancy, the pool becomes a familiar environment for labour, whether used at home or in a hospital.
- Floating in water relieves pain.

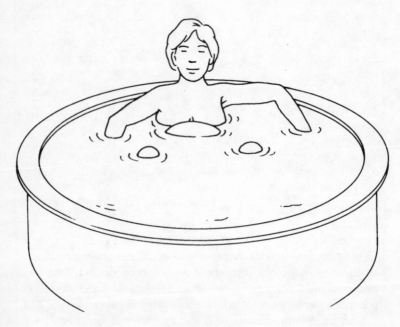

Figure 12 A birth pool

- Moving about in water offers comfort by relieving pressure on one's posture.
- During the later stages of labour, it may help a mother to let go of anxiety and tension.

The mother can give birth in the pool; providing skilled help is available there is no danger to the baby. Immediately after the birth, the mother should lie down, and a cool, wrung-out towel should be placed over the lower abdomen. This encourages the release of afterbirth materials from the womb.

CASE STUDY: MATERNAL BIRTH INJURY – 2nd *degree tear*

Sarah, aged 40, a psychologist, with a partner

Sarah had successfully given birth in a pool and on examination was found to have a second degree tear to the perineum.

Examination
The perineum is the 'floor' of the pelvis and is subject to intense strain during childbirth. The vagina may tear on delivery and when this is slight it is termed first degree. A second degree tear involves skin and underlying muscle.

Although casually considered to be a feature of birthing and sometimes created surgically, loss of continuity at the perineum is an injury. As such, it requires injury management – cooling, containment, elevation and rest – if it is to heal satisfactorily. Sarah's tear was extensive and bleeding but, understandably, having just given birth, she had no sensation of pain in her perineum. The attending midwife's offer to provide stitching was declined.

Treatment
A cold water compress was placed beneath Sarah's pelvis, brought up securely between her legs and laid across her abdomen. It was renewed after transfer from the delivery room to a recovery bed and remained in place while Sarah rested. This procedure allowed a cool compression to contain the injury.

After five hours, she had no bleeding from the wound and she was able to walk and urinate without pain before returning home.

She immediately went to bed and a new compress was applied. She continued lying down for the best part of three days, ensuring that the injury was elevated and free of pressure. The tear was uniting towards the vagina but the skin was unsealed.

The compress was used throughout the week and Sarah rested as completely as possible. Urination and defecation were without incident. Eight days after giving birth, the tear was healed.

Comment

Simply stitching a birth tear is inadequate. Undoubtedly, comparable injury to any other part of a mother's body would be considered serious. Failure to apply rudimentary first aid, risks adhesions, distress and unnecessary complication to future births. Using this hydrotherapy Sarah experienced no pain at all from her tear.

Osteoporosis

Porosity or the softening of bone tissue occurs in the middle, compact layer of bone, which is that part designed to bear the body's weight. This condition is not exclusive to women but since cases tend to occur from around the time of menopause, the suspicion is that the withdrawal of female hormones may predispose women to osteoporosis. The condition is characterized by discomfort, stiffness, nerve irritation and vulnerability to fracture.

Because of the powerful imagery of osteoporosis, sufferers unavoidably have a sense of a 'crumbling' skeleton, which causes anxiety and tension. Presently treatment involves mineral supplementation and hormonal therapy.

A major dietary study conducted by American researchers in China found osteoporosis to be uncommon even among the aged population. Chinese people consume only half the amount bone-hardening calcium that Americans do but they get it from vegetable sources. Moreover, women begin menstruating up to six years later in China and rarely develop serious reproductive disorders.

Considering that bones are supposed to be the second most durable body structure, osteoporosis in mid-life is curious. The Chinese study tends to confirm naturopathic observations that a diet rich in animal foods which promotes rapid growth in early

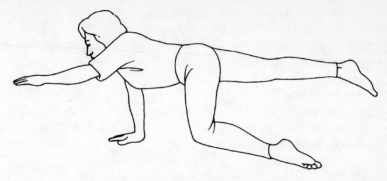

Figure 13   Begin graduated physical exercise which will strengthen bone by gentle stressing

life may increase the risk of premature degeneration, especially if the person is physically inactive. Taking all factors into account, naturopathy approaches osteoporosis as a postural problem.

Treatment

- Immediately eliminate dairy products from your diet and increase your intake of calcium-rich vegetables. It is almost impossible to overconsume food from vegetables sources.
- Do not take calcium supplements. Minerals are more easily absorbed from a wholefood.
- Have your neck and limb muscles massaged to improve mobility.
- Begin graduated physical exercise such as yoga movements, which will strengthen bone by gentle stressing.
- Become familiar with the structure of the skeleton and visualize its elegant framework to replace negative images of bones.

NATUROPATHY FOR MEN

Arterial Disease

Diseases of the heart and blood vessels are the leading cause of death of men in the UK and many other countries. Curiously, the heart's own blood vessels, which are privileged to receive the freshest oxygenated blood under the most impetus, are more at risk from damage than those at the periphery of the body.

There is general agreement that the major cause of cardio-vascular disease is poor blood supply. This is a result of inflexibility, brought about by fatty deposits on the walls of the arteries. Rigid arteries conduct blood less efficiently and have restricted blood flow.

Studies from around the world suggest that the build-up of fatty deposits can be prevented. Where fruit and vegetables play an important part in the diet, such as in France, the incidence of heart disease is low. Also, male populations in Greece, Italy and Spain, where there is a high consumption of the other known impediment to blood flow, tobacco, are believed to be protected from heart disease by generous fresh food intake.

It is not surprising since expressions such as 'heart attack' and 'my heart almost stopped' are in common use, that important life events appear to influence heart disease. Other research has shown that emotional reactions to events may be more important than the events themselves. Naturopathy suspects that a double protection exists in the emotional flexibility of male culture in southern European countries. Men can be shown to consume a more balanced diet but also may be less inclined to 'harden their hearts' emotionally than those in northern countries.

Cardiovascular disease is thought to be progressive. Warning sign are given in raise blood pressure, breathlessness and nervous sensations in the chest. This latter symptom, known as angina, is thought to be experienced equally by men and women. Yet far fewer women progress to serious heart disease. The implication is that men choose to ignore warning signs. Indeed, in one rehabilitation group for men who had suffered heart attack, it transpired that many had survived two or more incidents.

Dr Dean Ornish, an American physician, has developed a successful, fully documented programme for protection against and recovery from heart disease, which concurs with naturopathic practice.

Treatment

- If you are a northern European or American male (even if by default, having moved to those parts of the world), positively acknowledge the possibility of cardiovascular disease.
- As a matter of urgency, adopt activities which facilitate emotional expression, for example, paint, write poetry, join a choir – experience the risk of showing excitement and sadness.

- Eat fruit and vegetables at the start of meals every day.
- Avoid fatty foods, not only those from animal sources but any food which has been in refried oil.
- If you are a smoker, consider giving up.
- Only drink alcohol with meals.
- Have massage and learn how to massage.

Slipped Disc

Incapacitating low back pain is so common that by forty-five years of age, few men have not experienced it. At its most severe the sufferer is unable to move at all, while in milder forms discomfort extends from the back to the leg or groin. Popularly known as a 'slipped disc', the sensation which accompanies the onset of back pain is often described as 'something going'. Chronic back pain can lead to severely restricted movement and loss of confidence – the 'bad back'.

Humans' upright posture has been blamed for low back pain. Indeed no other animal is capable of bearing its weight on two legs for extended periods of time. However, humans did not simply rear up on their hind legs overnight but evolved the unique musculature which has enabled precision tasks to be done by the arms and hands. Also, studies done in developing countries show that the body is capable of withstanding greater physical strain without injury than experience in the West suggests.

It may well be that it is the sitting rather than the standing posture which contributes most to back pain. Normal seating, regardless of back support, places the weight of the body on the base of the spine for lengthy periods. Not only is this undesirable but it is further complicated by crossing the legs and collapsing the upper back, as the body attempts to relieve pressure. This is readily confirmed during a back-pain episode, when it is extremely uncomfortable to sit down.

With the exception of degenerative conditions which may affect the structure of the spine, naturopaths observe that much low back pain is essentially a muscular response, working in the patient's longer-term interests.

Unexpressed emotions are probably the most simple explanation of back spasm where no structural explanation exists. Neurological tests reveal that the lower back contains the greatest resting muscle tone of any area of the body. As nervous tension rises throughout the body, therefore, it is not surprising that the lower back can be brought into spasm.

There is also a tendency, possibly more common to men, for those who seek to maintain an rigid attitude towards people and circumstances to hold conflicting emotions back. The lower back may then become a convenient place to store the grimace, the clenched teeth and the furrowed brow which are not given a natural outlet. It is noticeable, however, that when low back pain sets in, it is very difficult to prevent expressions such as these returning to the 'front'. Viewed this way, the back is not behaving 'badly' but helping to circulate emotional energy.

Although advice is commonly given about how to use the back, lifting movements involve the whole body's muscles. Techniques or exercises which focus solely on the back muscles tempt strain.

While nerves may come under pressure and spinal joints become inflamed, the feature of low back pain is muscle disorder. Conventional treatment oscillates between bed rest and struggling on regardless with the aid of pain-killing medication. Naturopathy strikes a balance between rest and movement and enlists the support of massage and manipulation.

Treatment

- By the time a back 'goes' it is already undergong the body's own treatment. It is not necessary to panic. Pain is requesting that you lie down.
- Get as near as possible into the first-aid recovery position. Lying on one side will feel easier than on the other.
- Make contact with a practitioner you know (low back pain is so common, it worth establishing a contact now).
- Treat low back pain like blood-loss. With the practitioner's help get comfortable; do not be in a rush to get back to normal routines.
- Have frequent short (five minute) hot baths. Rest on your back with pillows beneath your knees; sleep on your side with a pillow between your knees.
- Do not attempt to stretch until you are completely pain-free. Walking, which is a gentle form of wriggling, is the best movement for the back muscles.

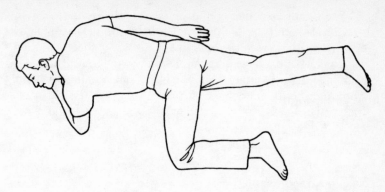

Figure 14   The recovery position

• Low back pain can be a warning of other, easily adjusted, pressure disorders. Discuss this with your practitioner.

CASE STUDY: *LOW BACK PAIN – incapacitating*

Tom, age 45, single, an actor

Tom was rehearsing for the lead part in a Shakespearean play when he suffered a fall and injured his lower back. He was removed to hospital for X-ray, which revealed no structural damage, but he was admitted. Treatment consisted of pain-killing medication and a support corset to immobilize the back. Tom was in a great dilemma, since he was anxious to play the role but he was also in pain. He was fearful that in attempting to do so he might injure his back further or break down during performance.

The theatre company consulted a naturopath and Tom was brought for treatment two days before the first performance.

Examination
Tom said that his overwhelming desire was to act in the play. However, his lower back muscles were in deep spasm and he had difficulty walking. At the first consultation it was not possible truly to assess the extent of his injury since he had also become very inflexible from being in bed.

Deeper examination found that Tom's pelvis was locked in rotation on one side of his lower spine. The pelvis normally makes a constant, rocking rotation to each side of the spine when walking. This explained the protective spasm throughout his back, making his vertebrae appear like a solid column of bone. The thigh bones are connected to the spine via the pelvis, so walking becomes limited. Added to this, the largest of the spinal nerves exit from this area so there is great sensitivity to pressure. Tom was doing well to be standing up at all.

Treatment
The treatment focused on Tom's desire to get through the first night of the play rather than 'mend' his back. Because a scene required him to take a fall and climb a staircase, a message was sent to the producer suggesting an alternative.

Tom was shown how to lie down using pillows to create a neutral posture, so that the act of breathing would have a gentle massaging effect. He was then shown how, by regressing to an 'all fours' position, he could move around much more freely. Feeling easier and in less pain he began to recover confidence in his body. Since standing upright was still very strenuous, a walking stick was given for support.

At the second treatment, friction massage was given to Tom's back and drainage movements made around the pelvis. From this it was possible for him to be moved more in the horizontal position. A gentle counter-rotation unlocked the pelvis and deep tension was released. He was shown how to apply strong contraction of his abdomen to 'corset' the pelvis from within and use this in conjunction with the stick to walk a little more.

The third treatment took place on the afternoon of the play's first night. Tom had deeper friction and drainage massage and mobility tests confirmed that the pelvis was correct. His upright movements were still cautious but his facial expression, which is a reliable guide to the state of overall tension, indicated that the state of his back muscles had improved. A relaxed expression of the brow and jaw muscles reflect looser shoulders and decreased spasm of the lower back. On the basis of this, traction was applied to further loosen the muscles. It was done with Tom in an upright position, hanging and swinging gently over the back of the practitioner.

Tom felt so improved that he suggested that he try a modified fall. Success reinforced his sense of recovery and he left positively for the first night.

Comment
Tom performed without difficulty and impressed all by taking the fall and climbing the staircase as originally planned. In discussion later with the practitioner, he was able speak about how feeling very 'wound up' about the part may have contributed the circumstances of his injury.

His recovery from the injury was swift, given the extent of the inflammation. As an actor he may have been unconsciously utilizing the power of visualization, which is known to have therapeutic potential. It is particularly useful when pain or shock creates disassociation from the body, as happened to Tom.

NATUROPATHIC CARE OF OLDER ADULTS

Rheumatoid Arthritis

The term 'arthritis' means 'inflamed joint'. It is used to describe painful swelling which restricts movement in the joints of the arm and leg, although it can also occur around the facets of the vertebrae (spondylitis).

These joints are cleverly constructed to allow for maximum flexibility, which is intended to last a lifetime. The spinal joints may begin to stiffen with age – probably from sitting – but free movements of the limbs can be found in people of advanced age. Yet rheumatoid arthritis, sometimes to a disabling and disfiguring degree, is very common throughout the Western world.

The inside of the joints is protected by lubricating fluid and the bones themselves are lined with a buffering material. If a joint is subject to constant pressure or used unnaturally (in the rotated hip position of classical ballet, for example) the bones may be subject to premature wear and tear. This condition, which is less common than the rheumatoid type is called osteo-arthritis.

While the factors causing osteo-arthritis are understood, those leading to rheumatoid arthritis are obscure, despite the fact that a great deal of research has been done, and there is evidence suggesting that the condition is unique to the human species.

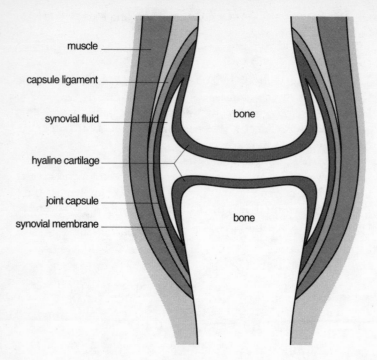

muscle

capsule ligament

synovial fluid

hyaline cartilage

joint capsule

synovial membrane

bone

bone

Figure 15   Cross section of a joint

What is known is that women appear to be more affected than men and the incidence in northern Europe is the highest in the world. The rheumatic joint is intact within its lubricating capsule, but the inflammation extends to the structures around the joint. The muscle ends which pass over the joint are principally affected, and the increased heat attracts an internal 'hydrotherapy' resulting in swelling.

Conventional theories about the cause of rheumatoid arthritis have come and gone with fashion. At one stage, when 'infection' held sway, sufferers might have their teeth, tonsils and appendix surgically removed. Later on, mega-doses of painkillers were advised, until gastro-intestinal side-effects became evident. At the moment rheumatoid arthritis is described as an auto-immune disease, in which for reasons as yet undiscovered the body chooses to attack itself.

Much as this latter suggestion goes against the grain of naturopathy's 'intelligent body', practitioners find an echo of causality in the 'self-destruct' notion. However, naturopaths observe that it is not the system which is in conflict but the individual. In structural terms, the muscles which pass over the joint work in opposing paired units, whose synchronicity ensures smooth articulation. This muscular choreography is termed antagonism. When muscular tone is uneven to the extent that joints are being moved under pressure, rather like wheels with brakes applied, they become hot from friction. Therefore, the inflamed joints of rheumatoid arthritis are really the side-show of the actual condition, which is chronic tension.

The question then arises as to how such tension could develop unnoticed. Naturopaths observe that it is often because the individual feels disempowered by fear from directing the tension outwards towards an external antagonist, be it a parent, a partner, an employer or the government. Raw tension is then converted into resentment, which is much easier to feel but not display. The energy of such resentment is easily taken up by initially supple muscles but eventually it inhibits articulation and in that sense may be described as an auto-immune condition: 'self attacking self'.

Wide-ranging studies have shown that rheumatism is aggravated by dietary factors, in terms both of ingredients and of eating patterns. Clinical findings show that anti-nutrients such as alcohol and tobacco smoke and high protein consumption tend to increase the inflammatory reaction, while eating too quickly, eating late at night and using food for solace are also implicated.

Sportspeople sometimes find that the site of an old injury can develop rheumatic tendencies. This is due to improper management in the rehabilitation stage. If an injured joint is used before it is sufficiently healed, a low-level inflammation will persist. In later life this can be irritated by a fall or twist and will manifest as a rheumatic-type swelling. This can be helped by hydrotherapy.

Treatment
- Since it is impractical within normal social convention to direct all tension outwards, keep the body moving in times of conflict.
- Rheumatoid arthritis is most common in the hands and feet; become aware of unconsciously clenched hands or curled toes.

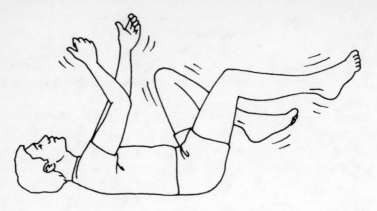

Figure 16   Indulge in a tantrum

- Combining the above two points, indulge in a tantrum when you feel frustrated by outside circumstances: lie in bed and beat the mattress with your fists while kicking up and down until you are breathless.
- Restrict your intake of animal-sourced protein foods. Eat slowly. Use raw foods and salads for controlled biting activity. Drink only a small amount of alcohol, in the company of others.
- If a joint swells when you are tired, it is likely to have been injured and not treated appropriately at some time. Seek naturopathic advice.

Rheumatoid arthritis is not predestined, nor is it an indication of the wear and tear of life, but rather of retreat from life. Persevere with the treatment. Numerous cases show that swelling may be arrested and mobility regained, even if symptoms are advanced.

6

Naturopathic Care of Children

At least 95 per cent of the ailments children are prey to will heal themselves. Paediatricians spend most of their time treating parental distress. The child rarely needs treatment but gets it anyway and is subject to its consequences, and it is the parent who gets the relief.

Dr Robert S Mendelsohn, leading US paediatrician

ORTHODOX MEDICINE IS inclined towards 'protecting' children's health via mass medication, but naturopathic care of children is more interactive, encouraging an exposure to life, while ensuring that a child's natural defences are built up from within.

Children are not 'little adults' but adults being grown. Compared with life in later years, childhood is a much more experimental, flexible and robust transition than many adults are able to recall. Anyone who has closely followed the typical day of a child will observe an eagerness for constant physical and emotional involvement which would exhaust even a teenager.

The intensity of childhood is reflected in the often dramatic nature of common childhood illnesses. Naturopathy finds a child's wholehearted physical commitment to the sudden fevers, breathing distress or refusal of meals which characterize early illnesses confirming rather than threatening. It is generally accepted that unless they are accompanied by serious malnutrition, the majority of children's illnesses are normally self-limiting. Naturopaths contend that these illnesses are associated with a child's efforts to exercise the eliminative organs and are firm that they should be allowed full expression.

IMMUNITY

Naturopathy finds the conventional concept of immunity by vaccination dubious and illogical, for many reasons. First, it is a practice which has more in common with superstitious ideas about disease concerning malevolent entities than modern, sophisticated medical thinking. Secondly, given biomedicine's fixation with methods for denying microbial entry to the body, the direct introduction of foreign material into the bloodstream is inconsistent. Thirdly, mass immunization is based on the assumption that everyone experiences disease in the same way, yet doctors are being encouraged to practise biomedicine with regard to the individuality of the patient. Fourthly, it inaccurately portrays immunity, a term whose correct usage implies that a direct, limited exposure to an experience raises our capacity to *endure* a similar but greater experience. Vaccines are promoted on the basis that they enable us to *avoid* the experience of a disease.

While individual substances are required to be tested for safety, no tests are done on the combined effects of vaccines. Because of this and since vaccination perpetuates the view of illness as the enemy, naturopaths do not support the vaccination of nourished children. For information on reservations about mass medication within conventional medicine, see the titles on child health in the Recommended Reading section.

For parents, the notion of vaccination is appealing, given that there are many influences on their child's health over which they have no direct control – the environment, heredity, birth circumstances and accidents – which may give the impression that an apparently defenceless child has need of immediate medical protection. This has to be offset against the fact that the materials which make up the child's body are millions of years old! Furthermore, most mothers have a resource which all opinions are unanimous in declaring to be the child's real passport to a healthy existence – breast milk.

BREAST MILK – THE PERFECT FOOD

It seems extraordinary that it has to be said that breast milk is the obvious food for a baby, but since the first days of hospitalized births, there has been tremendous pressure to give babies 'balanced' manufactured food. Since being hospitalized can be an intrusive experience for both mother and baby, it is understandable that for many breastfeeding is unsuccessful. It is not helpful, for example, that birthing practices such as separating mother and child immediately after delivery for relatively unnecessary procedures, delay contact with the breast. Despite thousands of years of human breastfeeding, it has taken less than a hundred years of hospitalized births to disrupt and often negate a child's ideal start in life.

Nature has arranged that breastfeeding is beneficial for both mother and child. Immediate suckling has been shown to prevent post-birth complications and assist in the reformation of the womb. In the longer term, the mother's weight tends to stabilize, and other findings suggest that breastfeeding reduces the likelihood of serious breast disease.

A baby's early feed is unique and contains ingredients which are clearly designed to complement its immune system and which may confer other benefits as yet undetectable. The nutritional composition of breast milk is perfect microbiologically, its temperature renders it perfectly digestible and a breastfed baby regulates its own consumption. Formula baby foods are cumbersome in contrast, and because they use ingredients intended for other animals, are suspected of introducing toxins to the baby.

SOLID FOOD

Naturopathy recommends that breastfeeding be extended well into the first year of a baby's life. There are two clear reasons for this. First, a baby may just be able to swallow foods within a few months but little will be digested. The appearance of one or two teeth does not confirm that a baby can begin chewing. Rather it will suck hard on a solid and may cause deformation of the upper palate, which can result in nasal obstruction. Solid foods are sometimes given to babies because they seem to encourage sleep. This is because the intestines' requirements for blood temporarily deprives the brain. Not only is this inferior sleep but it may set up a cycle which results in a tired, irritable baby.

Secondly, giving concentrated foods to a baby's premature digestive system is thought to produce intolerance to these foods in later life, seriously disrupting nutrition. The introduction of lightly mashed fruits and vegetables at around the ninth month will ensure that a baby makes a smooth transition to a full diet. Thereafter, food as and when the child is hungry – whole-grain starchy foods for energy and lacto-vegetarian proteins – adequately provides the required nutrition.

Children recognize the emotional power of food early on – its comfort value, its fun and its potential for mischief-making, and their conscious attitude towards individual foods are unlikely to be based on nutrition. So while stressing the importance of balanced meals, naturopaths suggest avoiding confrontational situations with diet. Children's creativity and inventiveness will extend to food, perhaps resulting in wild swings of preference or revulsion and, occasionally, quite harmless over- and underconsumption.

Early eating behaviour – its quality, quantity and attitude – determines the dietary habits of a lifetime.

CHILDREN'S ILLNESSES

Since in effect a baby is a 'product' of its mother and father, it will inherit not only the parents' external characteristics but also their systemic constitutions. A recognition of this should restrain biomedical treatments being imposed upon children, especially in earlier years when their eliminative systems are seeking to establish their individuality. If this is repressed by medicines then, according to naturopathy, the child is in effect destined to suffer the illness patterns of its parents.

Needless treatment is not harmless; it has a tendency to escalate symptoms. Self-limiting conditions can be complicated by reactions to invasive tests and procedures. More lastingly, medicalization contributes to the polarization of symptoms into an organic category separated from emotional life. It is not surprising, therefore, that by adulthood some individuals are unable to cope emotionally after being so fundamentally disconnected.

Reassurance

The naturopathic view is that children's treatment needs to be balanced with long-term benefits. When it is thought to be necessary to consult medical opinion for a serious illness, it needs to be remembered that while a clinical intervention may produce an immediate effect, the responsibility for maintaining the health of a child belongs to the parents. At these times, consultation with other parents or grandparents is especially recommended, for often parents' real concerns can be confused with fears of the unknown.

Reassurance filtering down to an ailing child creates a healing effect and has the power to distinguish whether treatment is appropriate or necessary.

Emotional Security

That children use their parents as role models from earliest times is graphically demonstrated by comparisons of their posture. Even in a family whose members have been separated for many years, boys invariably stand and walk like their fathers, while daughters can, in remarkable detail, copy the posture of their mothers. This is most noticeable when a child is brought in for naturopathic consultation. Since practitioners work with the understanding that posture reflects emotion, when presented with a child in emotional difficulties the symptoms are clear: whichever way the emotions work in the family, it is not working for the child.

By 'acting first, considering later', children reveal that part of the interior, ancient human brain where life is either secure or not, with no grey areas. When a child's behaviour reaches disturbing levels – beyond an adult's tolerance – it is understandable to want to stop it, even if this involves restraint. Unfortunately, this sends a confusing signal to the child, who more often than not is reacting to an insecurity. Learning to understand the meaning of compromise is part of a child's development, but naturopathy does not believe that this should come in the form of medical treatment.

Practitioners observe many disorders which appear to be associated with the suppression of emotional problems. These include breathing and eating difficulties, sleep irregularities and in particular, skin disorders. A disturbed child's skin clearly and obviously conveys signs such as 'angry', 'weeping' or 'cracking up'.

While treatment is being directed towards unpleasant physical symptoms, emotional energy may become focused on less direct 'targets' in a child's social life, further complicating the situation. As is often the case, not until the physical symptoms themselves show resistance to medicines and become a further cause of distress, are children likely to be offered emotional help. It is an unfortunate feature of conventional medicine that even when problems are acknowledged from the outset to be of emotional origin and deemed psychiatric, literally meaning 'of the soul', treatment is invariably pharmaceutically based.

Insecurity is at the centre of a multitude of children's emotional problems. It is best treated by the concern and attention of their nearest and dearest.

CASE STUDY: EARACHE *'infection of the ear'*

Claire, aged 10

Claire felt a 'cold' coming on over a few days and was put to bed. During the night her temperature increased and she was disturbed by earache.

Examination
Consultation took place by telephone with Claire's parents, who had experienced naturopathic treatment.

Inflammation of the mucous linings in the head is so common that a medical speciality exists to treat it – ENT, standing for ear, nose and throat. The majority of cases are children and naturopathy accepts that this should be so. The eliminative linings in the head are conveniently near major body exits and are constantly, if invisibly, helping to relieve potential toxicity. Compared with devitalized adults, children are vigorous in their need to eliminate and heightened activity is usually accompanied by dramatically raised temperature. For some children, the ear is the most painfully affected area. The structure of the ear is such that even slight congestion increases pressure, and aching ears are more likely to create an overall headache than is a congestion of the nose or throat.

Conventional medicine is alert to the danger of serious ear conditions but naturopathy believes that medicalizing acute ear disorder as an infection is mistaken. Controlled studies show that medical treatment is ineffective and may be potentially harmful.

Treatment
Claire was immediately given cool foot baths to relieve the pressure in her head. Foot bathing works through 'revulsion', whereby the circulation is temporarily distracted from congested blood vessels. Unlike the treatment of external injury, it is not advisable to put cool cloths directly over systemic inflammation. Foot baths were recommended twice daily or when the pain returned. A warm, dry cotton towel was used against the ear to increase comfort.

Claire was not hungry. Since heat created by the digestive process tends to aggravate raised temperature and lead to discomfort, her parents were reassured that fruit or juices were appropriate.

Simple massage of the shoulders was offered and deep mouth breathing was done when Claire felt able to. Within a few days, her ears felt near normal and she returned to a lightening cold.

Comment
Claire's parents found the foot bathing particularly useful in coping with her illness. They felt that Claire steadied from that point and they gained confidence in the treatment. They noted that although the episode seemed to be exhausting her, she emerged clearer and stronger.

The aim of naturopathic care of children is to minimize interference. The vast majority of childhood illness are known to be self-limiting. So necessary are they for a child's system, they normally run their course regardless of outside intervention. Simple hydrotherapies, dietary adjustment and reassurance can effectively relieve discomfort and provide useful distraction. Anxious parents are advised to seek naturopathic treatment.

7

Naturopathic First Aid

*Water has a therapeutic power in so far as it is a catalyst to our
need to survive. The need to survive and the process of healing
are part and parcel of the same thing.*
    Dr Michel Odent, internationally-acclaimed obstetrician

FIRST AID IS AN urgent response and its aim is threefold – to
preserve life, prevent a condition worsening and promote
recovery. Life is threatened because many disturbances are
experienced by the body as a shock, and delicate, homeostatic
mechanisms are challenged. Further complications can be limited
by timely first aid and through reassurance and containment, and
this in itself provides circumstances favourable for a satisfactory
recovery.

Naturopaths recognize that appropriate first aid is often the
most important aspect of healing. An example of this is the need
to contain a wound by limiting movement in its early stages,
otherwise adhesions may develop. Adhesions arise when layers of
injured tissues become stuck together following irritation. They
can cause lifelong discomfort, even though the initial injury
apparently heals well. Irritation can also be produced by certain
foods and by anxiety, so naturopathic first aid encompasses a
wide range of responses to an injury.

Injuries may be defined as trivial or serious. Trivial injuries,
such as slight bruising or small cuts, often go unnoticed and
disappear within 24 to 48 hours. Serious injuries are much more
disruptive and involve more bleeding. Since it is not always
possible to determine the extent of an injury judging by its cause
alone, assessment should be made quickly according to other
obvious physical signs. The most important signs are the amount

of blood lost (although be aware that the bleeding may be internal) and the reaction of the patient.

HYDROTHERAPY

Naturopathic first aid is based on an understanding that an injury or wound is a form of trauma and that treatment should involve physical and psychological support. Because of its physical properties and emotional associations, water, in the form of hydrotherapy, has traditionally been the first aid of naturopathy.

Since the human body takes its form within a watery environment, it should not be surprising that contact with water is conducive to healing. If there are misgivings concerning hydrotherapy, however, they are almost always based on misconceptions about its methods and application. The first is invariably about moisture being associated with fungus – in fact this condition only arises from moisture being trapped around the skin. The second is that cold water is 'shocking' to the heart, whereas very hot water, which is often used in a bath, has a much greater potential to shock the circulatory system. There are also irrational attitudes towards water which may have to be considered – if a person has had an unpleasant experience from choking or bathing, water may have threatening associations.

Hydrotherapy was developed in 19th-century Europe from techniques used in folk remedies. Vincent Priessnitz is credited as the pioneer in the field, but the most famous early hydrotherapist was Sebastian Kneipp, a Bavarian priest. Kneipp avoided an early death by embracing hydrotherapy, and later became an internationally renowned healer. Kneipp's followers have succeeded in bringing the traditions of hydrotherapy into the modern era, and there are numerous well-documented examples of its effectiveness in pain relief, as a reliable sedative and in the restoration of healthy circulation.

It is not difficult to explain how hydrotherapy works. Being warm-blooded, the human body benefits from contact with cool water; briefly applied, the water acts as a tonic, while extended application has a calming effect. Contrasting hot and cold water is also used and occasionally, longer hot applications. Hot hydrotherapies are versatile in that they can be anti-inflammatory when placed in opposition to an injury.

The benefits of hydrotherapy are:

- Cold water limits bleeding in the easily damaged small blood vessels. Although ruptured capillaries constrict spontaneously, cold helps to restrict pressure from nearby vessels by reducing blood flow. This is useful since the walls of blood vessels instantly begin to repair after being damaged.
- Cold water reduces the pain of pressure or inflammation. The peripheral nerve endings are almost immediately desensitized by the application of cold. There is a split-second sensation, then the nerves gradually lose feeling. Hot water must never be used on an injury, since it would encourage bleeding.
- Cold water is reassuring. If the local application is complemented by a cool cloth to the neck or forehead, the casualty will relax and breathe more easily, feel more confident, and be less likely to lose consciousness.
- Cold water keeps the injury supple. Often it is necessary for a casualty to move or be transported. As this might further irritate the wound, cold water stops it drying out, preventing the injury from being irritated.
- Cold water encourages elimination by relaxing the skin. Even if debris is deposited deep within a wound, it will be pushed up by the deeper layers of the skin as long as the surface is kept moist.
- Alternating hot and cold water provides a gentle massage effect. The first pressure on an injury should consist of alternate hot and cold, which will encourage drainage, reduce pressure and relieve discomfort. If it is free of pain an injured part may then be gradually moved.
- Hot water is able to redirect the flow of blood from congested areas. This is especially useful with a wounded limb. Applying heat to the uninjured side attracts the blood and reduces pressure towards the injury.
- Hot water is reassuring in the later stages of first aid. While warm water is relaxing generally, locally applied heat is contra-indicated within twenty-four hours of injury. A short warm bath thereafter eases muscle tension and may assist sleep.
- Water is ecological and economical. Water supplies are normally clean and plentiful and hydrotherapies do not require that water is microbiologically sterile. The most important aspect is relative temperature: 'hot' need only be a little above blood heat and it is unnecessary to add ice to produce 'cold'.

Methods

Almost any form of injury, from simple bruising to maternal birth injury, can be helped by hydrotherapy. The method of application depends on the area to be treated.

The influence of hydrotherapy is initially recorded in the skin and then distributed around the body via the nervous reflexes and circulatory routes. The water is administered by various methods, ranging from splashing to immersion, as well as from moist compresses. Hydrotherapies are suitable for people of all ages and are particularly valuable for children, who both benefit and actively enjoy the treatment. The methods generally used in first aid are:

- immersion – injuries to the extremities are placed under water as soon as possible. Where the skin has been cut or torn, water is allowed to flow over the opening before pressure is applied
- compress – the skin is covered by a damp piece of cotton or linen, covered by a thicker dry material such as wool
- splashing – a spray is run over joints or inflamed areas

Apply cold water to an injury using any method until experienced help arrives.

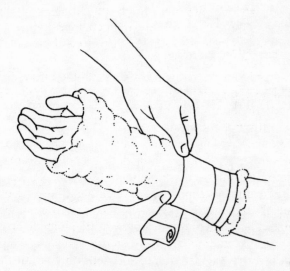

Figure 17   A compress

FASTING

A casualty is may feel thirsty, and can be given small sips of water, but it is unlikely that food will be requested. In fact, it is likely that anything that has been recently consumed will be ejected by the body. Naturopathy recommends that, as in the case of acute illness, a casualty should not be encouraged to eat a full diet until real appetite returns. Juice fasting during the early painful stage of an injury has two advantages:

- The blood's white cells are not distracted from repair and cleansing activities at the injured site. Complex foods passing through the digestive tract always claim the priority attention of the white cells.
- Although eating often seems to reduce pain from the injury, after food has begun to be digested, the return of full circulation to the injured site increases discomfort.

Neither 'energy' foods such as starch and fat nor 'building' ingredients such as proteins are useful to the injured body. Energy for the restoration of the body is probably taken from stores within the liver. However, a diet of fresh juices or vitamin- and mineral-rich raw fruits and vegetables ensures adequate nourishment. As appetite returns, small amounts of starch and protein can be reintroduced but if the injury again becomes painful, a juice fast is recommended.

Eat a full diet only when free of pain.

CASE STUDY: *MALIGNANCY* – '*Cancer of the Mouth*'

Alan, aged 60, single, a singer

This is an exceptional case in that it is not strictly a first-aid report and it has not been possible to follow up this treatment. However, it does illustrate fasting as a response to an emergency. Alan made an emergency appointment. He had earlier been to see a specialist at hospital, who had diagnosed a malignant growth in his mouth. Immediate radical surgery had been recommended. Alan was set against having surgery not only in principle but because he had taken exception to what he felt had been a dismissive style of consultation. He quoted the specialist as saying, 'Surgery or you'll be dead next week.' Instead, he proposed that he fast on juices for thirty days and asked for naturopathic supervision.

Examination

On examination Alan was found to be reasonably fit for his age. He had a mild skin rash and some joint stiffness, and was slightly fatigued. He did, however, have an almond-shaped pink mass towards the rear of his upper palate.

The practitioner had reservations about such a long fast, especially as it was midwinter and Alan lived alone. Alan said that he had some experience of shorter fasts and on the basis of this was going to go ahead, with or without supervision. An agreement was reached that the practitioner would collaborate with Alan provided that he telephone the practice at the same time on the same day each week. If he failed to call in, then the practitioner would telephone to advise against continuing.

Alan did call in each week as planned, and sounded well, if a little subdued. After twenty-one days, although he did not actually feel hungry, he had begun to fantasize about food, so he decided to terminate the fast.

When he presented for his next visit, he was a leaner, calmer and altogether younger version of his former self. On examination, he had improved in every respect. His skin condition had cleared up, his movements were relaxed and he said he felt very well. The mass on his palate was slightly reduced.

Alan intended to maintain a vegetable diet. He discussed his plans to return home to Tasmania shortly but said he would contact the practitioner before leaving. He never did. Three months after the second appointment, the practitioner saw Alan walking along the street. He was moving fast enough to be overtaking other people and was soon out of sight.

Comment

There are many aspects of this case which are not possible to verify. Perhaps Alan's growth was misdiagnosed; perhaps he did not really fast; perhaps he fabricated the entire episode. But if it is true, his case illustrates two important findings about response to malignant disorder.

First, we have suggestions from psychological studies of cancer conditions that 'fighting the disease' is not enough, and that long-term survivors possess a strong reason to get well. In Alan's case, he gave the impression that he was indignantly determined not to die the following week or for a very long time, more so than he was afraid of having cancer.

Secondly, recent research has tended to vindicate fasting, by clearly showing that drastically reducing food intake boosts the body's production of hormones. These chemicals provide protection against the development of cancer cells and appear to be depressed by overeating.

Alan gave every reason to believe that his self-treatment had been successful in the short term. It is not possible say more than this. Perhaps he might come across this book, recognize his case study and re-establish contact with the practitioner.

SUPPORT

An injured animal makes for the nearest place of shelter and security and lies quietly until it is healed. Human beings, who lead a more pressurized social existence, have devised plasters, bandages and plaster of Paris to maintain a dignified conviviality when injured. This 'sectioning off' is often to the detriment of healing, since overactivity accompanied by tension may cause the injury to recover incompletely or, as often in the case of damaged joints, become a site of low-level inflammation in the future. Simple body movements with regular deep breathing will provide the injury with much-needed oxygen.

Naturopaths observe that injuries are often associated with times of disintegration in the casualty's life. It can therefore be regarded as a form of communication, even if only a self-transmission. It is therapeutic, therefore, to regard all injuries as serious from the casualty's point of view and offer maximum support.

Any injury to a particular tissue – a cut in the skin, a torn muscle, a fractured bone – will evoke a response in the whole body. The effect on a wider area of the body than the focus of injury is evident in swelling, inflammation and stiffness. The lymphatic system is stimulated and nodes between the injury and the chest may become enlarged and sensitive. Although the injured part will normally be immobilized and supported, support should also be offered to the whole body for as long as possible.

Physical pain is an expressed emotion – failure to recognize the personal seriousness of injury not only encourages premature activity but may also provoke another injury. First aid is inadequate without reinforcing emotional affirmations along the lines of 'You are going to be all right', accompanied by touch or eye contact. False positive statements such as 'It's only a . . .' or 'Don't cry', deny the experience of the injured.

Have body massage to maintain emotional integrity while injured.

LOSS OF BLOOD

Although the body is capable of making up a small loss of blood, the circulatory system is strained by a loss beyond 0.5 litres. Even a small amount of bleeding should be restrained by pressure, although simply raising the injury above the level of the heart can be equally effective.

Shock

A major loss of blood produces shock, a reaction whereby the body goes into full autonomic mode – pupils become dilated, the skin is cold and clammy and the pulse is faint but rapid. This often occurs where bleeding is internal, from a fall or pressure injury. The main aim in cases of suspected shock is to keep the patient conscious, elevate his/her legs above chest level and summon an ambulance immediately.

It is always wise to despatch a casualty to hospital if blood loss has been great or if evidencing a state of shock. However, even for a trivial injury, the casualty should be observed for twenty-four hours.

THE SKIN

The commonest first aid situations involve the skin, perhaps in the form of bruising, laceration, cuts, punctures, burns or stings. Since the cosmetic aspect of treatment is very important in skin healing, and because naturopathic treatment is usually outstandingly successful for such injuries, it is worth giving a detailed first-aid profile for the skin.

Contrary to its superficial appearance, the skin is very lively organ. Organs are highly organized parts of the body and foremost in the skin's activity is defence. It is also very regenerative, which means that under favourable circumstances it rapidly reproduces itself. However, because the skin is intimately connected to the functioning of the other organs of the body – the kidneys in particular – first aid should be extended beyond the surface.

An examination of the skin shows that it is constructed of a deeper layer, known as the corium, which is rich in blood vessels and nerves resting on a supple cushion of fatty cells. From this extend microscopic structures which are responsible for its delicate eliminative functions, such as heat loss. The skin is also capable of retaining heat and of synthesizing vitamin D from the effect of sunlight on it. Attached to the corium is the visible membranous covering of the skin, called the epidermis. It is this part of the skin which sometimes 'peels' or, when very dry, scales off as 'dandruff'.

Because of its interface with the environment, the skin is probably the most robustly defended part of the body. This

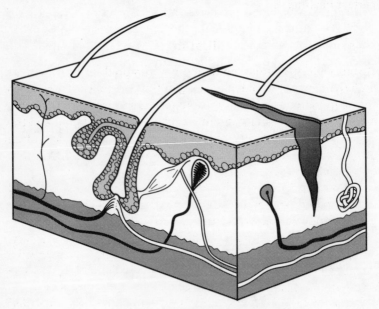

Figure 18   The layers of the skin

robustness is even thought to allow the skin to share the strain of other parts, for example in relieving pressure on the nervous system and helping eliminate digestive disorders.

It is an important feature of naturopathic treatment generally that the body be allowed to express its disorder into the environment, rather than have it suppressed because of a phobia about germs. The fear of external contamination is best illustrated in orthodoxy's well-meaning but naturopathically premature closing up of an injury by sealing over the epidermis. The scarring which often results is almost entirely absent in the naturopathic method. Given the skin's anatomy of growing from the inside out and its outstanding defensiveness, it seems over-reactive and illogical to attempt to close up its damaged surface chemically or mechanically.

First aid to the skin is akin to conditions in the womb. A reconstructive surgeon working on congenital abnormality has commented: 'From the moment babies are delivered, wounds scar. In the womb they heal perfectly.' In life outside the womb, amniotic fluid is replicated by the body in the formation of a blister over a skin injury. Using hydrotherapy, naturopaths aim to give injuries this watery advantage in promoting perfect healing.

Bruising

A bruise forms after capillaries are ruptured in the skin or underlying muscles. Blood escapes and is seen collecting beneath the skin, after which it is drained back into the returning circulation. The water content is reclaimed by the blood and the cell debris is eventually eliminated. Bruises are tender, often lasting some days, and are accompanied by local stiffness. Sometimes bruises 'come out' later, after injury and may be confusingly distant from the site of an impact, since gravity will draw free blood downwards. Easily bruised skin suggests an unbalanced diet and water retention in cells.

Bruising belongs to the relatively trivial category of injury, except where a bruise continually reappears from a repetitive impact at work or from sport. Here the capillaries may become irritated, weakened and eventually lose function. It is not desirable in the long term for any tissue to suffer repeated irritation because of the likelihood of escalating inflammation.

Treatment

Treat with a cold-water compress. Wring out a piece of cotton or linen, 1 inch wider than the bruise on either side, in cold water and wind it once around the body over the bruise. Wind a length of wool, like a scarf, wider than the cotton, on top. Reapply the compress when it becomes dry or three times per day until the stiffness is relieved. Do not wear it at night.

Laceration

This occurs when the skin is torn and may range from a graze to the detachment of a sizeable piece of skin. Skin which is lacerated downwards or horizontally has a poorer circulation, while upward lacerations have a greater chance of retaining tissue. Pieces of skin should always be left attached to the body. Lacerated skin will bleed freely, which initially helps cleanse the wound but needs to be stopped quickly by a cold application. The surrounding area will be infused with lymphatic material and the skin will feel tight. If it occurs on the lower limb, walking may be uncomfortable.

Deep laceration may leave disfigurement of the skin, so hydrotherapy's cosmetic advantage is very important.

Treatment

Support the skin with a cold piece of cotton and pour cold water over it for two minutes. Apply a cold-water compress as for bruising. Replace the compress with a fresh piece of cotton as soon as it begins to dry out (the deeper the injury the sooner this will be). If the skin becomes dry it will tighten and irritate the lacerations.

The compress should not be used overnight. Before bed, the whole area should be held under running water to be cooled and a dry cotton covering put in place. If during the night the injury feels painful, this can be repeated. Compressing may continue until fresh skin is evident over the injury, which may take up to seven days.

Incision

An incision may be a cut from a kitchen knife, a stabbing or even the insertion of a surgeon's scalpel. Simple cuts heal quite spontaneously, such is the skin's defensiveness. The main problem with an incision is that even within the clinical atmosphere of the operating theatre, foreign material may be deposited beyond the skin's normally impenetrable defences. Should this occur, a reaction will take place, which is usually termed an infection. Nearby lymph nodes will become active. Whereas the orthodox view is that this is a sign of a war between the body and an infectious agent, naturopathy contends that it is the natural behaviour of the skin to eliminate unwelcome matter.

Although stitching and dressings can artificially draw together the edges of an incision, naturopathy prefers to allow the skin to re-form slowly from its deeper layers. This allows the easy exit of foreign matter and lessens scarring. (If the edge of a wet linen compress is placed within a contaminated cut, it may be left in and will 'grow out' retaining debris.) Incisions can also be very painful, since nerve endings can be severed and are even more painful during recovery. It is also very important to restrict the movement of a deep cut to avoid adhering tissues.

Treatment

An incision should be held in running water for two minutes. Deep cuts may not bleed profusely as larger vessels tend to constrict spontaneously. A firm cold compress should be applied and the area immobilized by a bandage. Often the casualty will be in shock so precautions should taken against fainting, including a cold cloth to the back of the neck. The compress should be renewed to keep the cotton continually wet but should be removed overnight and cooled as for a laceration.

An incision may take from seven to fourteen days to repair but sensations of itching around the wound confirm that healing is well established.

Puncture

Although the injury may be small, a puncture wound can be irregular, depending on the force with which it occurred. It may be further complicated by fragmented parts remaining embedded within the skin. Using hydrotherapy, it is possible to avoid the distress of debridement – the removal of foreign bodies by further excision. With effective compressing, debris will naturally arrive on the surface of the skin.

Treatment
The wound should be immersed in cold water for fifteen minutes. Apply a soft cotton compress lightly. Keep the wound moist by changing the cotton frequently. Remove the compress at night and cool the wound. Each morning immerse the injury for fifteen minutes before fresh compressing. As the wound will be free of pain, allow fourteen days before considering surgical removal of any debris.

CASE STUDY: *SKIN INJURY – with lacerations and puncture*

Margaret, aged 60, married, a grandmother

Margaret had fallen full length onto a path. In breaking her fall with her hands, she had cut into the skin and pieces of tarry stones had become embedded in the palms. She was treated with an antiseptic skin salve and bandaged. The stones were to be removed later at the surgery. Her hands were very painful.

Examination
The hands were swollen and inflamed. The salve had sealed over the cuts.

Treatment
Thick cotton cold water compresses were applied to her palms and they were rebandaged. Her hands were immediately less painful and remained so for the duration of the day. Dry bandages were applied overnight.

Fresh compresses applied in the morning were changed in the late afternoon. The first compress was seen to be stained by tar. Gentle wrist movements were advised to assist drainage. This hydrotherapy was continued for seven days. As it was removed, each compress was found to have tarry debris from the wound.

By the seventh day, the palms were pink and clear. No discomfort had been felt since the second day of treatment.

Comment
The patient gained confidence in this treatment from the outset since it provided immediate pain relief. Success meant that the foreign materials did not have to be removed surgically from the skin.

Burn

Burns respond very favourably to hydrotherapy but speed of recovery depends on their depth, size and location. In addition, a burn is categorized according to severity: *first degree* burns are red and swollen and painful but without blistering: *second degree* burns are deeper, more painful and have blisters; *third degree* burns involve destruction of the skin's superficial layer, without blisters, although coagulated veins may be observed. The thinner skin of children and older adults suffers greater injury from burns.

Apart from skin injury, serious burns deprive the body of fluid. The 'rule of nines' can be applied to decide whether a burn requires hospitalization. This states that a surface area of the body equivalent to one limb represents 9 per cent of the total. A 5 per cent second degree burn requires hospitalization. The treatment described here is intended for first degree burns and second degree burns that are less than five per cent. As a guide, hot liquids give more superficial injury than contact with flames or prolonged contact with hot objects.

Treatment
Cool the burn rapidly with flowing water for ten minutes. Apply a linen compress to keep the injury constantly moist, which ensures effective pain relief. It is likely that a burn will initially dry the compress quickly so it needs to be renewed often. If the linen becomes attached to the skin, it need not be removed but can be simply resoaked. If a hand, elbow or knee is burned, it should be bandaged to prevent the skin being stretched. Compressing keeps a burned area supple and encourages smooth re-growth of the skin.

Stings and Scratches

Stings or scratches can be very serious, depending not only on the injury but on the casualty's allergic reaction. Sensitivity to this type of injury may be increasing since many allergy-provoking substances are appearing in the environment.

Treatment

A bee sting should be scraped from the skin and a cold compress applied until it is comfortable. A sting to the mouth or throat should be treated by sitting in a cold bath. Scratches should be cooled then cold compressed. Reaction to stings and scratches may involve a lymphatic response, so the nearest lymph nodes may be cooled.

First aid is offered as the best available help to the injured until expert assistance is obtained. The response will vary with each individual casualty, especially people with arterial disease, diabetic conditions or nutritional deficiency. Well-tested naturopathic first aids, based on physiology and sound experience, are safe, even in the hands of the inexperienced.

8

Taking Naturopathy Further

ALTHOUGH THERE ARE signs that naturopathic philosophy is beginning to infiltrate modern health-care concepts, it will take time to influence practices in the conventional hospital and consulting room. But because of its practicability, and the trend towards greater self-involvement in health care, it is possible to gain benefits from naturopathy immediately.

BY ONESELF

Since naturopathy is essentially self-care, it has a reliable history to encourage application of the principles outlined in this book – perhaps not all at once but as circumstances present, for example using hydrotherapy on an injury or experimenting with a juice fast when feeling 'off colour'. From these experiences, conviction in the healing processes of the body will grow. For some people this will be an almost mystical realization, while for others, merely refreshingly obvious. Healing oneself can lead to positive changes in many areas of life because more energy is available once irrational fears about disease, or even about the body itself, are erased.

To help you follow up particular areas of interest in topics discussed in this book, an extensive list of books is given in the 'Recommended Reading' section. Although authors may stress differences in certain practicalities, this is because as a humane philosophy naturopathy is unavoidably infected with the person-ality of practitioners. In fact, for both patient and professional practitioner, a definition of naturopathy is not so much *what* is done, as much as *who* does it.

INFLUENCING MEDICAL PRACTITIONERS

Confidence in one's own healing tends to increase one's assertiveness. At the very least, being naturopathically informed should enable you to respond better to even the most antagonistic medical practitioner.

The clinicians cited in the 'Recommended Reading' section are well experienced in the application of naturopathy, many from over forty years' practice. Even if the resources of conventional care were available, the justification of the effectiveness of naturopathy in formal research terms is inappropriate. There is evidence from the number of orthodox authors listed, however, that the medically trained are still open to persuasion.

It is doubtful whether the intellectual argument for naturopathy impacts on biomedically trained doctors. However, from what has been written by naturopathic doctors, it appears that there is an appeal which may resonate ethically with ideals and ambitions which existed before their training. Often, less than ideal medical practice is excused by suggesting that doctors merely respond to the low expectations of patients. If this situation really does exist, loaning a doctor a copy of a book which has been helpful to the patient should improve the quality of care offered.

HOW TO FIND A NATUROPATHIC PRACTITIONER

Albeit few in number, fully professionally trained naturopaths are to be found throughout the world. In the English-speaking countries they may not have attended conventional medical school, whereas in Germany and India, naturopathy is integrated into conventional training. In the UK, non-medical naturopaths have complete freedom to practise and set up clinics; in parts of the USA, it is illegal to practise any form of medicine without a medical licence. Some doctors, having embraced the balanced Greek ideal, without embarrassing their colleagues practise medicine naturopathically.

Practitioners can be found in the telephone book or in registers available in local libraries. Those who publish are usually obliged to promote their work and can be traced through bookshops, libraries and via the Internet.

There is little danger in receiving naturopathic guidance but as levels of schooling vary, a clear idea of a practitioner's professionalism can be gained from information about their regulating body. This should contain details of the form of training and accreditation, as well as a code of conduct and procedures for complaint. Consultation with an unregulated practitioner is not recommended.

For many patients, a reliable route to treatment is personal recommendation of a practitioner by a friend. Yet because of the interpersonal nature of consultation, the success of this type of introduction is not guaranteed. Discovering a practitioner with the right 'feel' is important, so it is worth seeking out another contact if necessary.

LIVING NATUROPATHICALLY

There are institutions, centres and spas which offer treatment with extended accommodation, and which afford the opportunity to experience naturopathy fully. Here new rhythms can be established, deeper rest obtained and inspirational examples from others' lives shared.

In former times these places were often directed by the 'heroes' of naturopathic history and were infused with exciting, passionate atmospheres. No doubt much of their success with patients can be attributed to a pioneering energy. Dynamic practitioners contribute to a key factor in recovering health – helping to provide a reason to get well. Presently, although they are probably run more efficiently and professionally, residential health centres tend to have a more passive ambience, where serenity is a priority on the assumption that guests are 'worn out' and require sedation rather than stimulation. Alternatively, for those desperate about life and health, it is sometimes suggested that by taking oneself off to a wilderness and surrendering to nature, a state akin to naturopathy might ensue.

On the Aegean island of Skyros, in spectacular settings, there exist two holiday centres which, in eschewing extremes, have reincarnated the essence of naturopathy. Using classical Greek ideals, they offer a programme of land and sea activities, creative adventure and body–mind therapeutics. The staff act as assistants, facilitators rather than healers, and all participants come together to create a sense of community. The aim is to give guests a 'get away from it all' experience and enable them to return with new perspectives on 'real life'. The centres have been established for twenty years and, by all accounts, they have succeeded in meeting participants' needs.

BECOMING A PRACTITIONER

The discovery of naturopathy usually leads to improvement in energy, emotional poise and an optimistic outlook. Often a spectacularly beneficial experience of treatment leads someone to consider becoming a practitioner. It is not necessary to take a formal training to contribute a naturopathic influence – parents, teachers and politicians all have the power to interpret naturopathy for others' good. Many professional health workers such as psychologists or physiotherapists may be naturopathically inclined. However, since fully trained practitioners are rare or their work prohibited, naturopathy needs as many committed professionals as possible.

A practitioner's work may be interesting, demanding, reward-ing and frustrating – all in one day or even within one consultation! Treating the patient as well as the symptoms means that the practitioner's involvement is more than technical. There is every chance that the patient will ascribe the benefits of treatment to nature and themselves, while failure may be held to be the practitioner's fault!

Training schools exist in the UK, the USA, Australia, New Zealand and Israel. In European countries and India it is possible to take naturopathic studies alongside conventional medical training. Courses usually run for three to four years full time. Some individual naturopaths take on apprentice students, who receive tuition while assisting in the practice.

Practitioners are trained in the health sciences, nutrition and human behaviour. Most importantly, they attend clinical sessions where they learn how to listen for the spoken and unspoken clues which patients' symptoms offer.

Qualified practitioners can expect a busy career in private practice, depending on their level of commitment. Although naturopaths tend not to specialize consciously, many develop expertise in postural and nutritional areas, others in systemic problems, while childbirth and children's conditions offer great scope for naturopathic help. Health centres and spas also offer employment, but patients there are often drawn from a narrower section of society.

Most practitioners will be self-employed in English-speaking countries but there is a trend for practitioners of a range of complementary disciplines to work together in a group practice. This is a useful way to prevent a sense of isolation in the early days of practising and can also work for the benefit of patients, by utilizing case conferences and interdisciplinary meetings.

Recognizing the potential strain in intensive clinical work, many naturopaths choose to work part time, even when their practices become established. By complementing one-to-one work with lectures and related activities, there is less chance of the 'burn-out' associated with other forms of therapy.

Appendix

The Personagram

QUESTIONNAIRES IN 'HEALTH' MAGAZINES are popular, partly because they offer the reader an insight into the determinants of their health but also because they often give the possibility of a *response*. In some ways this is not unlike the naturopathic consultation. Naturopaths prefer to look into the patient's life for answers to problems rather than subject signs and symptoms of ill-health to investigative tests.

When symptoms persist despite biomedical or naturopathic treatment, however, they invite deeper understanding. For example, a few days' rest or a course of antibiotics is usually effective in clearing up the 'common cold'; persistent colds or a cold which reappears quickly suggests more complex symptoms. Similarly, we might require simple relaxing treatment for occasional aches and pains in our muscles and joints but the severity of strain which produces arthritis solicits a more profound approach.

THE LANGUAGE OF SYMPTOMS

Naturopaths treat symptoms respectfully as coded messages concerning issues in a patient's whole life. Although disturbing and often distressing, they provide alternative views from conscious perceptions. In this respect symptoms and night-time dreams are very similar, speaking as other selves as if to say, 'This is how the situation looks from our perspective.'

Patients whose symptoms are persistent or particularly troubling emotionally are encouraged to attempt to decode their

120

meaning by using a technique which has come to be known as the 'Personagram'. Similar versions are used in different cultures throughout the world where illness is not viewed as an isolated, accidental experience.

The idea of meaningfully conversing with different parts of oneself is considered unusual only in science dominated Western society. In other societies, a person may consist of many 'selves'. In the Zinacanteca culture of South America, for example, an individual has eight selves, each associated with a different body part. For Hindus in the subcontinent of India, an individual is regarded as having seven levels of manifestation.

In Western countries, individuals who overtly exhibit signs of communicating with other selves are deemed to be 'possessed'. A diagnosis of Multiple Personality Disorder ensures appropriate psychiatric treatment, usually in the form of benumbing medication. It is ironic, of course, that the physician may admit to a junior colleague to being in 'two minds' about exactly what type of treatment to use.

TECHNIQUE

Drawing from imagination, the patient materializes a minimum of three characters, real or fictitious, dead or alive, human beings or caricatures. Each character is given an identity and relationship to the others. On prompt by the practitioner, by extending their imagination the patient speaks spontaneously for each character. Note is taken of what is said for discussion later. Characters may also speak through gesture or be represented by painting or drawings.

This matter-of-fact description of the Personagram belies its powerful emotional impact. The technique begins rather superficially with the presentation of only three characters, especially in those who consider themselves as having 'no imagination'. As the characters begin to speak, however, an emotional connection is established and a rapport builds up. The 'conversation' continues until each character is satisfied with his or her contribution.

It is important to stress that the Personagram is a communication device and not a diagnostic tool. Users gain insight into their relationship with symptoms, which releases tension and recirculates energy. Patients are not given a sense of personal responsibility for inducing illness but an empowerment to initiate positive change.

The Personagram may be used for any symptom but is particularly useful when an individual has come to the 'end of the road' with treatment and begins to feel hopeless. It is also helpful when symptoms are frightening or begin to develop extensively, such as a skin condition, and to cause alarm. The Personagram utilizes the power of visualization, an exercise of the imagination known to produce therapeutic effects.

Stage 1

On a blank sheet of paper, write out approximately six lines describing character 1. Give them a name, age, marital status, nationality, etc., and other distinctive features. Say something about their interests or passions. Place them geographically in the world or within a room.

Repeat this for characters 2 and 3. Remember that characters may be real or imagined and do not be confined to everyday time and space – a character could live on the moon or have magic powers!

Do not be surprised if you feel slightly self-conscious at this stage, since the characters are actually emerging from your consciousness. And do not be disappointed if the characters appear predictable or somewhat uninteresting. Materializing three distinct entities is enough for the time being.

Stage 2

Now follows a series of questions or prompts which the patient answers on behalf of the characters. Responses should be spontaneous, 'off the top of one's head'. Make sure they are written down.

1 Ask each character any questions which would give more information about their personalities, e.g. happy or sad/secure or insecure.
2 Are the characters aware of the existence of each other? Are they connected in any way? If not, why not – e.g. 'not until now'.
3 Ask each character in turn if they have any difficulties in relating to the others.

4 Offer each character the opportunity to acknowledge or communicate with the others. This may take the form of approaching or distancing themselves physically; it may be by warmly embracing them or violently detaching themselves; it might be in a one-word sentence or a monologue.

5 Ask each character how they feel about the communication.

6 If you are working with a practitioner, a discussion will follow about whether you have any comment on using the technique. If you are working alone, spend a few minutes reflecting on any particular aspect which has left a strong impression. Be accepting and do not attempt to 'tidy up' the final scenario.

7 Keep a record of the Personagram.

Usually a patient experiences a heightened self-awareness after using the technique. Sometimes direct connection is established with a symptom, while at other times a general feeling of release from pressure is gained. Occasionally a patient will have a very vivid but not frightening dream within a few nights.

A Personagram can be repeated by developing original characters at a later date or new characters can be devised or added. Personagrams can also be used to prepare for stressful events or to reduce the strain of seemingly intractable situations.

Glossary

acute illness of rapid onset and usually short duration.

adhesions sticking together of body linings as a result of irritation.

Asclepius Ancient Greek god of medicine, son of Apollo.

allergy a reactive condition of the body, from organic or emotional stimulus.

allopathy treating illness with drugs which oppose the action of symptoms.

antibiotic a drug used to combat infection, which works by interfering with the formation of a bacterium but may also disturb normal body cells.

antidepressive a drug used in psychiatry to treat mood disorder.

anti-inflammatory a drug which suppresses inflammation to relieve pain.

Ayurveda the indigenous medicine of the Indian subcontinent.

biomedicine medical practice which regards expression of illness as biological malfunctioning.

blood pressure a measure of the pressure at which the heart pumps blood into the large arteries. 'High' pressure signifies strain within the system; 'low' pressure is associated with dizziness and disorientation.

cardiovascular relating to the heart and the blood vessels.

case record the record of investigation of illness and treatment programme devised.

chronic illness of long duration and degenerative change.

complementary the holistic system of medicine which embraces the original Greek ideals of Hygieia and Asclepius.

consultation the forming of a relationship from the meeting of the consultant and patient.

corticosteroids hormones formed in the cortex of the adrenal glands which control inflammatory responses; often given in the form of synthetic drugs to suppress inflammation.

elimination actions of the organs which are designed to expel material unwanted by the blood.

empathetic a type of co-feeling, which enables a practitioner to offer detached but compassionate support to the patient.

epidemiology studies done on large populations which chart the course and trends of diseases over long periods.

fasting abstaining completely from foods or consuming only juices.

frictions massage strokes which relieve stiffness without deep pressure.

Hippocrates born 460 BC, the 'patron saint' of holistic medicine: 'Life is shaped by our search for food and congenial surroundings – medicine should be an extension of that search.'

homeostasis the constancy maintained within the body despite external fluctuations eg temperature.

hunter-gathering prehistoric humans' way of eating, which relied principally on plant foods.

hydrotherapy the external use of water for treating injury and illness.

Hygieia Ancient Greek goddess of health, daughter of Asclepius.

hypertension high blood pressure estimated to cause damage to the body.

iatrogenesis illness inadvertantly caused as a result of medical intervention.

infection entry into the body of bacteria which multiply and cause poisoning.

interstitial fluid the fluid space between the body's cells.

lacto-vegetarian a diet of plant food, eggs and milk products.

lymphatic the secondary circulation of the body which returns the fluid escaping from the blood at cellular level.

massage rhythmic movements performed by hands or feet which relax, condition and stimulate the body's functioning.

medicalization overextension of biomedicine to treat all expression of symptoms as biologically based.

mobilization applied movements which help restore flexibility to the body.

motor nerves nerves which transmit activating messages to muscles.

mucous membrane the slimy protective and eliminative surfaces of the body's linings eg in the intestinal tract or bronchial tubes.

nutrition the process which involves food digestion and respiration, resulting in the maintenance, growth and repair of the body.

parasympathetic nervous activity beyond conscious control which helps calm the organs.

percussion massage strokes which raise muscular tone and stimulate blood circulation.

pharmacology the study of the action of drugs and their effects on the body.

predisposition an underlying condition which makes for susceptibility to illness or injury.

psychiatry biomedical specialization for treatment of mental and emotional disorder.

rehabilitation a treatment programme which aims to re-establish functioning and fitness after injury or illness.

self-limiting illness eliminative illness which 'runs its course' regardless of medical treatment.

sensory nerves nerves which carry information from organs, especially the skin, back to the brain for processing.

signs physical evidence of illness, eg a rash or swelling.

stress intolerable pressure on the nervous system, which produces acute symptoms.

sympathetic nervous activity beyond conscious control which stimulates the organs.

symptoms subjective experience of illness – 'I feel pain/distress.'

Tai Chi graceful choreographed exercise which forms part of traditional Chinese medicine.

tone a harmonious state of tension within the body.

traction to relieve compression on a joint but especially on the spine, by gentle stretching.

trauma an injury which results in body discontinuity and shock.

treatment therapy which complements natural body functioning.

unconscious beyond conscious control.

unprocessed in a natural state, not subject to adulteration.

yoga a system of physical, mental and emotional practices which help maintain spiritual well-being.

Recommended Reading

Bircher, Ruth, *Eating Your Way to Health*, Faber, London, 1961

Buchman, Dian Dincin, *The Complete Book of Water Therapy*, Keats, New Canaan, Conno, 1994

Bythman, Joanna, *The Food We Eat*, Michael Joseph, London, 1996

Dries, Jan, *The New Book of Food Combining*, Element Books, Shaftesbury, 1995

Eaton, S Boyd, Marjorie Shostack and Melvyn Konner, *The Stone Age Health Programme*, Angus & Robertson, London, 1989

Fulder, Stephen, *How to be a Healthy Patient*, Hodder & Stoughton, London, 1991

Glouberman, Dina, *Life Choices, Life Changes*, Thorsons, London, 1989

Helman, Cecil F, *Culture, Health and Illness*, Butterworth–Heinemann, Oxford, 1994

Jack, Alex, *Let Food be Thy Medicine*, One Peaceful World Press, Becket, PIA, 1991

Kennedy, Ian, *The Unmasking of Medicine*, Allen & Unwin, London, 1981

Kirchfeld, Friedhelm and Wade Boyle, *Nature Doctors*, Buckeye Naturopathic Press, Ohio, 1994

Ledermann, Erich K, *Medicine for the Whole Person*, Element Books, Shaftesbury, 1997

McKeown, Thomas, *The Role of Medicine*, Blackwell, London, 1979

Mendelsohn, Robert S, *Confessions of a Medical Heretic*, Contemporary Books, Chicago, 1979

— *How to Raise a Healthy Child . . . in Spite of Your Doctor*, Ballantine Books, New York, 1984

Menninger, Karl, *Man Against Himself*, Harcourt, Brace & Co, New York, 1938

Mitchell, Stewart F, *Health Essentials: Massage – A Practical Introduction*, Element Books, Shaftesbury, 1992

— *The Complete Illustrated Guide to Massage*, Element Books, Shaftesbury, 1997

Nichols, Keith, *Psychological Care in Physical Illness*, Croom Helm, Kent, 1984

Odent, Michel, *Water and Sexuality*, Arkana, London, 1990

Ornish, Dr Dean, *Programme for Reversing Heart Disease*, Ballantine Books, New York, 1996

Price, Weston A, *Nutrition and Physical Degeneration*, Price-Pottinger Foundation, LA Mesa, CA, 1979

Scheper-Hughes, Nancy and Margaret M Lock, *The Anthropology of Affliction: Critical Perspectives on Medical Anthropology*, Free Press, New York, 1997

Shelton, Herbert, M., *Health for the Millions*, Natural Hygiene Press Inc, Connecticut, 1968

Sidenbladh, Erik, *Water Babies*, A & C Black, London, 1983

Thomson, C Leslie and Alec Milne, *Nature Cure Monographs*, Kingston Publications, Edinburgh, 1994

Thomson, Jessie, *Natural and Healthy Childhood*, C W Daniel, London, 1976

Van Straten, Michael and Barbara Giggs, *Superfoods*, Dorling Kindersley, London, 1990

Watkins, Alan, *Mind-Body Medicine: A Clinician's Guide*, Churchill Livingstone, Edinburgh, 1998

Wittkower, Eric D and Hector Warnes, *Psychosomatic Medicine: Its Clinical Applications*, Harper & Row, New York, 1977

Useful Addresses

Australia

Australian Natural Therapists Association (ATNA)
PO Box 308
Melrose Park
South Australia 5039
Tel: 61 8 371 3222
Fax: 61 8 297 0003

Federation of Natural and Traditional Therapists (FNTT)
238 Ballarat Road
Victoria 3011
Tel: 61 3 9318 3057

Canada

Canadian College of Naturopathic Medicine
60 Berl Avenue
Toronto
Ontario M8Y 3CY

Europe

British College of Naturopathy and Osteopathy
Frazer House
6 Netherhall Gardens
London NW3 5RR
United Kingdom
Tel: 0171 435 6464
Fax: 0171 431 3630

General Council and Register of Naturopaths
Goswell House
2 Goswell Road
Street
Somerset BA16 0JG
United Kingdom
Tel: 01458 840072
Fax: 01458 840075

Incorporated Society of Registered Naturopaths
Kingston
Edinburgh EH16 5UQ
Scotland

The Skyros Centre and Atsitsa, Greece
Administration:
92 Prince of Wales Road
London NW5 3NE
United Kingdom
Tel: 0171 267 4424/248 3065
Fax: 0171 284 3063

USA

American Association of Naturopathic Physicians
2366 Eastlake Avenue East
Suite 322
Tel: 206 323 8510

or

American Association of Naturopathic Physicians
PO Box 20386
Seattle WA 98112

American Naturopathic Association
1413 King Street
First Floor
Washington DC 20005
Tel: 202 682 7352
Fax: 202 289 2027

Index

Page numbers in **bold** *refer to the glossary.*

acute conditions 21–2, **124**
adhesions 100, **124**
adults 72–92
Africa 3–4, 32
alcohol 75, 91
Alexander technique (AT) 33–4
allergy 75, 113–14, **124**
allopathy 39–42, **124**
angina 84
antibiotics 11, 15, 21, 40, 120, **124**
antidepressive drugs 41, **124**
anti-inflammatory drugs 40, **124**
anxiety 37–8
appetite loss 23–4, 38
arm and leg treatments 62
arterial disease 83–5
arteries 64
arthritis 19, 33, 37, 89–92, 120
Asclepius 8, **124**
asthma 33, 75–7
attachment 38–9
autonomic nervous system 51
Ayurveda 8, **124**

babies
    learning from 29–32
    see also breastfeeding; children

back
    lower back massage 36
    lower back pain 32, 85–9
    treatments 60, 61–2
biomedicine 1–2, 10–11, **124**
    attitude to life and death 43–4
    and the 'child' within 73
    for children 96
    diagnosis and labelling 19–20
    and emotional expression 39
    and emotional symptoms 4–5, 41, 98
    illogicality of treatment 21
    impact of the 'fringe' 12–13
    influencing practitioners 116
Bircher-Benner, M O 29–30
birth pools 80–1
birthing 78–82
blood 52
    loss of 107
blood pressure 4, 37, 79–80, **124**
bones 32–3, 57, 82–3, 89
brain 66–7
brain stem 67
breastfeeding 4, 29, 94–5
breathing 35, 75–6
    and chewing 30
    in treatments 53–4, 63, 66, 76–7, 99
bronchioles 75–6
Brookes, Tim 26

bruising 109–10
burns 113
Bushpeople (!Kung) 3–4
butter/margarine controversy
    28–9

calcium 82, 83
cancer 11, 14, 31
    of the mouth 104–6
cardiovascular system 11, 83–5,
    124, *see also* circulatory
    system; heart disease
case records 48–50, **124**
cerebellum 67
cerebrum (cerebral cortex) 67
chewing and breathing 30
Chi 8
'child' (within the adult) 73–4
children 93–9
China 8, 11, 82
chronic conditions 22–3, **124**
circulatory system 64–6
comfort eating 31, 56
complementary medicine 13, **124**
consultation 47–50, **124**
conventional medicine *see*
    allopathy; biomedicine
corium 108
corticosteroids 31, 40, **125**

death *see* life and death
degeneration 11, 22–3
dental health 4
dependency 38
diet *see* nutrition and diet
digestive system 30, 22, 51–6

earache 98–9
eczema 21
Edren, Lennart 32
electro-convulsive therapy (ECT)
    41
elimination **125**
eliminative systems 21–2, 69–71

emotion 36–9
    allopathic treatment 41
    and asthma 75–6
    and digestion 56
    and elimination 70
    and food 29, 31, 96
    and heart disease 84
    and lower back spasm 85–6
    and pain 42, 107
    and rheumatoid arthritis 91
    security in children 97–8
    see also psycho-physiology
empathetic 47, **125**
endocrine system 51–4
epidemiology 11, 27, 73, **125**
epidermis 108

fasting 31–2, 104–6, **125**
fear of dying 44
first aid 100–14
food manufacturing industry 28,
    29
fresh foods 29–30
'Freudian slips' 38
frictions **125**
'fringe' medicine 11–13

Gadamer, Hans-Georg 46
Germany 12, 116
glands, swollen 21
gorilla behaviour 31
Greece, early 7, 8
Greenock, Gavin 31

haemorrhoids 33
heart 42, *see also* cardiovascular
    system; circulatory system
heart disease 14, 23, 83–5
Hindus 121
Hippocrates 7, 29, **125**
homeostasis 1, **125**
hormones 52
hospices 44
hunter-gathering 3–4, **125**

hydrotherapy 101–3, **125**
  first aid treatments 110, 111,
    112, 113, 114
  other treatments 63, 64, 66, 69,
    70, 71, 77, 78, 79, 81–2, 99
Hygieia 7, 8, 11, 13, **125**
hypertension 4, 37, **125**
  in pregnancy 79–80

iatrogenesis 12, 74, **125**
immunity 14, 15, 94
incision wounds 110–11
India 8, 11, 116, 121
indigestion 22, 30, 54–6
infection 27, 40, 44, 70, 73, 90,
    125
  'ear infection' 98–9
'injury proneness' 37
interstitial fluid 64, **125**
invigoration treatments 62–3
irritable bowel 37

joints 19, 32, 57, 89

Katsuyne, Professor and Mrs 30
Kearney, Ray 31
kidneys 69–70, 108
Kneipp, Sebastian 101

laceration wounds 110
lacto-vegetarian proteins 96, **125**
large intestine 30, 69–70
Latto, Gordon 12
leg and arm treatments 62
Lief, Stanley 12
life and death 43–5
lifestyle 72–7
living naturopathically 117–18
Lock, Margaret M 1
lordosis 36, 77
lungs 69–70, 75–6
lymphatic system 64–6, 106,
    125
  swollen glands 21

massage 35–6, **125**
  in treatments 54, 59, 61–3, 66,
    68–9, 70, 79, 83, 85, 88, 99
McKeown, Thomas 17, 27, 43–4
medicalization 96, **125**
men 83–9
Mendelsohn, Robert S 93
metabolism 30, **125–6**
Middle Ages 9
mobilization **125**
  in treatments 59, 60, 68, 88
motor nerves 60, 67, **126**
movement 15, 18, 32–6
mucous membranes 70, 77, 98,
    126
Multiple Personality Disorder 121
muscular system 33, 60–4, 85–9

naturopathic practitioners
  becoming 118–19
  finding 116–17
neck region treatments 59–60
neurological (nervous) system 42,
    66–9
nutrition and diet 4, 15, 17–18,
    27–32, 51–2, **126**
  and asthma 75
  and heart disease 84
  and osteoporosis 82–3
  recording 49
  and rheumatism 91
  in treatments 56, 66, 71, 77,
    78, 83, 85, 92

Odent, Michel 100
older adults 89–92
one health, one disease principle
    19–20
organs 50–1, 108
Ornish, Dean 84
Osler, Dr 9–10
osteo-arthritis 22, 89
osteoporosis 32–3, 82–3
overweight 54–6

pain 42–3
painkillers 43, 90
parasympathetic nerves 22, 36, 67–8, **126**
percussion **126**
perineum, torn 81–2
period pain 77–8
Personagrams 120–3
'phantom' pain 42
pharmacology 10, **126**
posture 18, 32–6
    assessment 50
    children's 97
predisposition 37, 126
pre-eclampsia 79–80
pregnancy complications 79–80
Price, Weston 27
Priessnitz, Vincent 9, 13, 101
processed foods 27, 28, 29
proteins 49, 91, 92, 96
psoriasis 21
psychiatry 19–20, 121, **126**
psycho-neuro-endocrino-
    immunology (PNEI) 14–16
psycho-physiology 4–5, 18–19, *see also* emotion
puncture wounds 111–12

Raynaud's syndrome 21
reassurance 96–7
refined carbohydrate 28
rehabilitation **126**
relaxation treatments 63–4
respiratory system 51–4
rest 15, 23–4, 70, 71, 80, 81–2
rheumatoid arthritis 89–92
Rikli, Arnold 9, 13

salt 4, 28, 49, 75, 77
Scheper-Hughes, Nancy 1
scratches 113–14
self-care 115
self-limiting illness 93, 96, 99, **126**

sensory nerves 60–1, 67, **126**
shock 107
signs 20, **126**
sitting posture 33, 60, 85
skeletal system 32–3, 57–60, 82–3
skin 21, 42, 69–70, 97
    injuries to 107–14
Skyros holiday centres 117–18
sleep 24
slipped disc 33, 85–7
smoking *see* tobacco and smoking
solid food (introducing) 95–6
southern Europe 84
speaking out 38–9
spondylitis 89
sports injuries 37, 91
stings 113–14
Stockholm marches 31–2
strain 33–5
stress 22, 31, 36–7, **126**
    and digestion 22, 37, 56
support 106–7
sympathetic nerves 36, **126**
symptoms **126**
    allopathic treatment of 1–2, 39–42
    friendliness of 20–1
    language of 120–1
    predisposition to 37–8
Systems Theory of behaviour 4–5

Tai Chi 69, **126**
Thomson, James 12
tobacco and smoking 22, 84, 85, 91
tone 60–1, **126**
traction 59, 60, 88–9, **126**
trauma 101, **127**
treatment **127**
typhoid 10

unconscious 61, **127**
unprocessed foods 29–30, **127**
USA 11–12, 116

vaccination 15, 94
vagus nerves 68, 69
varicose veins 33
vegetarian diet 52
veins 64
visualization 89, 122

women 77–83

yoga 35, 54, 62, 77, 78, 83, **127**

Zinacanteca culture 121